THE HEART OF CARING

THE HEART OF CARING

a life in pediatrics

MARK VONNEGUT, M.D.

SEVEN STORIES PRESS

NEW YORK • OAKLAND • LONDON

SEVEN STORIES PRESS
140 Watts Street
New York, NY 10013
www.sevenstories.com

College professors and high school and middle school teachers
may order free examination copies of Seven Stories Press titles.
Visit https://www.sevenstories.com/pg/resources-academics
or email academics@sevenstories.com.

Library of Congress Cataloging-in-Publication Data

Names: Vonnegut, Mark, author.
Title: The heart of caring : a life in pediatrics / Mark Vonnegut, M.D.
Description: New York, NY : Seven Stories Press, [2021]
Identifiers: LCCN 2021035222 (print) | LCCN 2021035223 (ebook) | ISBN
9781644211052 (hardcover) | ISBN 9781644211069 (ebook)
Subjects: LCSH: Vonnegut, Mark--Health. |
Pediatricians--Massachusetts--Boston--Biography. | Sick children |
Physician and patient. Classification: LCC RJ43.V66 A28 2021 (print) | LCC RJ43.V66 (ebook) |
DDC 618.9200092 [B]--dc23
LC record available at https://lccn.loc.gov/2021035222
LC ebook record available at https://lccn.loc.gov/2021035223

Printed in the USA.

9 8 7 6 5 4 3 2 1

To patients, teachers,
and parents everywhere,

Thank you for letting me
have such a good time
when I go to work.

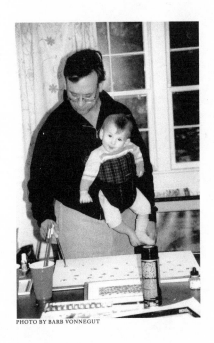

PHOTO BY BARB VONNEGUT

"Science knows no country, because knowledge belongs to humanity, and is the torch which illuminates the world."

LOUIS PASTEUR, M.D.

"Scientific work . . . must be done for itself, for the beauty of science, and then there is always the chance that the discovery may become, like radium, a benefit for humanity."

MARIE CURIE, PH.D.

CONTENTS

INTRODUCTION

I have had an absolute ball taking care of babies and children. There's no greater honor than having people trust me with their children. I'm afraid more newly minted doctors won't have the same choices, opportunities, and joy that I've had. I've been able to figure out how to take care of patients on my own terms, and it feels like getting away with something. When I tell medical students that I used to practice pediatrics for twenty dollars per visit, everyone paid cash, and three doctors shared one all-purpose employee, they think I must be talking about the dark ages. As things are, it's now doubtful that young doctors will be able to practice primary-care pediatrics in the same community for forty-plus years.

There was nothing romantic or outdated about how we ran our practice forty years ago: we provided accessible, affordable, very high-quality care and we made a living at it. I was able to pay back my educational debt in eighteen months. Because many of today's residents are carrying half a million dollars in educational debts, going into primary care pediatrics is financially risky and private independent office practice is going the way of the dodo. People assume that there must have been a lot wrong with the way we did things and that what's replacing us must be more efficient. Not true.

The job of the doctor is to take care of patients. We did a better job of it forty years ago. There was an assumption that doctors knew what they were doing and would ask for help if they needed it. That alone saved many billions of dollars. When we saved money it went back into patient care. Patient care was 90-plus percent of what hospitals and doctors did. Now, coding, billing, and negotiating with insurers make up about half of what hospitals do.

The reasons why doctors can't afford to go into primary care pediatrics, 30 percent of hospitals have gone bankrupt, and patients can't afford medications are the same. The money went elsewhere. Back when patients paid cash, they had more power. Medical care cost a fraction of what it does now. And doctors had a much better time. We worked harder and there was no burnout.

The cure for burnout is letting doctors and nurses treat treatable diseases. It is what we went to school for. It would be (and is) infinitely more expensive to do anything else.

Remembering how to ride a bike

> "Life is like riding a bicycle. To keep your balance you must keep moving."
>
> ALBERT EINSTEIN

I'm a seventy-three-year-old man, shaved, showered, and ready to go to work. When I set up the office I have now, I had a shower put in. I thought maybe I could ride a bike to work and take a shower when I got there. The shower never got used, and we had to rip it out to make room for a giant new refrigerator to store vaccines.

I drive a bright-blue Mini Cooper with white racing stripes, a good sound system, and an extra forty horsepower that can make the car fly even when I don't mean it to. Two years ago I was stopped for speeding, but the cop let me go without a ticket or even a warning. I had been his pediatrician.

I saw and still see science as a refuge from ambivalence and uncertainty. In the eyes of science we are all equal. Who's right and who's wrong are supposed to be settled by math and science, not by who has the most money and power.

Science and progress don't advertise; they just are, and they belong to everyone. In the struggle between the mission of medical care and the money of medical care, surely mission would win. How could it not? I still believe that to be true, even though money is currently winning.

Forty years ago, I rode my bike approximately five mostly flat miles along the Charles River to Massachusetts General Hospital (MGH), affectionately referred to as Man's Greatest Hospital (because that's what it happens to be), where I was an intern and then a resident. I always rode as hard as I could and passed as many other bikers as I could. There might have been a blizzard or two that forced me onto the MBTA, but for the most part I rode to work regardless of the weather. I was not just another father, husband, and homeowner trying to support my family and having to borrow money; I was a bike racer. Now, my oldest son rides his bike to work regardless of the weather; it must be genetic.

At the end of the ride I entered MGH's pediatric service, where we took care of the world's sickest, unluckiest babies and children. One important thing we learned was how to protect our patients from black magic, snake oil, and quackery.

Biking, sweating a little or a lot depending on the weather, I thought about meningitis, epiglottitis, sepsis, congestive heart failure, renal failure, cancer, cancer, cancer, failure to thrive, appendicitis. As interns we worked hundred-plus-hour weeks and slept at the hospital every third night in closets with creaky metal bunk beds. As junior and senior residents we worked a little less.

We were often able to save kids from illnesses that once were almost always fatal, like leukemia and meningitis. I remember the ones for whom we couldn't do much and the haunted look they had that seemed to say, "You could save the others, why not me?"

If there has to be such a thing as cancer, why do babies and children have to get it?

In 1979, the nurses, the doctors, the lab and x-ray techs, the receptionists, and everyone else at MGH shared the belief that we were doing good work, doing it well, and trying to do it better. It was freedom from the curse of ambivalence. MGH and other hospitals were independent entities. They could and did control what they did and how they did it.

We knew racism and inequality existed, that not everyone had access to Mass General and the other teaching hospitals where we were educated and trained, but we saw inequality as one more source of pain and suffering we were in the process of conquering.

When I thought about what things cost, poverty, and the other social determinants of individual or global health, it was with an underlying optimism that science and progress would lead to more science and more progress, which would benefit everyone. The collective "we" were all on the same page. No one refused vaccines.

"The greatest good for the greatest number." For myself and most other doctors back then, being a doctor was practically a religious calling. The contract we signed read something like, "I'll devote myself utterly and completely to science and the care of my patients. The collective 'you' will protect me from financial, political, and other forms of predation."

"Sorry I'm late, dear, I was snatching children from the jaws of disease, death, and disability."

During the fifties, we conquered polio for pennies and dimes, literally. We turned leukemia into a curable disease and invented chemotherapy. The average cost of a prescription was about ten dollars. What you needed to be evaluated in the MGH pediatric emergency room was a worried parent and a child with a symptom of some sort. The average cost of an ER visit was less than one hundred dollars. If you couldn't pay, you didn't get chased by collection agencies. There were no co-payments or deductibles.

When I was twenty-one in 1968, the average family paid approximately two hundred dollars per year for medical care, including doctors, hospitals, medications, and health insurance. This was possible because health insurance was a relatively new thing and most people didn't have it. Most healthcare was paid for out of pocket. No matter how sick or desperate they were, people simply couldn't afford thousand-dollar pills, ten-thousand-dollar ER visits, or million-dollar hospitalizations, so such things didn't exist. People have now "reformed" how medical care is paid for to the point that it is unaffordable for many and life expectancy is falling.

We had the March of Dimes and other medical charities, but the idea that there would be large bets placed by investors in hopes that they, personally, would reap enormous profits from medical innovations was unthinkable. Science belonged to everyone. It was about mission.

In the late seventies and early eighties, as medical students and residents, we saw patients as quickly and efficiently as possible without rushing them. To do anything else would have been disrespectful. The biggest challenge doctors face now is accepting the diminished scope and ambition of what they do. The medical care I learned about in medical school and as a resident is a million miles away. This is my story of how we got from there to here. Today's residents are barely in charge of when they go to the bathroom.

✦ ✦ ✦

Doctors, especially the ones who think they're slick and clever, are naive about money and business. Doctors assume that the rich and powerful will admire them and want to be friends with them. They like stock tips, get-rich-quick schemes, and poker. Professional gamblers and salesmen can see them coming a mile away.

"Hey, Doc, how's it going? Pull up a chair. I hear you went to Harvard. Nice. Pick a card, any card. I'm sure your luck is about to change. I can just feel it."

Grandiosity

On the Fourth of July, three years ago, I was admitted to McLean Hospital. Going crazy is easy. Getting better is hard. Bipolar disease and psychiatric hospitalizations have been a wild card in my life. I pray to God I'm done with psych hospitals. It helps to have something to come back to, like being a doctor or being an artist or musician. Or friends or family. For me, psychosis has always been about caring too much. How can you be a doctor and not care too much?

It was six months after my trip to Haiti and the Haitians working on my unit played a significant role in my recovery. They were amused and maybe a little baffled by my attempts to speak Creole and the fact that I liked hanging out with them. Lots of famous people, like James Taylor, have gone to McLean. I finally got into a place with some class, but it didn't really matter. Being acutely

21

psychotic is so overwhelming it blots out the sun. Among my other symptoms was a deep distrust of white people. About the only people I trusted were the Haitians who ran the kitchen and were night staff and janitors. Without Haitians, McLean and a lot of other hospitals, and the patients for sure, would be up the creek. The Haitians gave me their attention. It wasn't delusional to believe that they cared about me and helped gently bring me back to the planet Earth.

My Russian psychiatrist was less than worthless. I had one run-in with him after my wife, Barb, brought in a softer bed mattress for my back pain. He must have assumed the pain was part of my craziness, but it turned out to be a slipped disc compressing a nerve. When he refused to let me have the softer bed, I asked him, "Do you have a Hippocratic oath in Russia or do you just wing it and send patients who complain to Siberia?"

Thank God for Haitians.

Watch out for Russians.

It's not good for me to get too upset about what's happened to medical care over the past forty years, and I very much hope I'm done with psychosis.

What happened roughly a year before I became psychotic was that my practice, along with a lot of other practices, was forced to adopt a very expensive and truly horrible electronic medical record (EMR) system that was, in effect, part of a giant strip mining operation designed to scoop up as much money as possible as fast as possible.

It truly was terrible but not worth going crazy over, and going crazy didn't help. It was and is the way of the world. If our practice couldn't survive the hit, we'd have to fold up our tents and move on or become part of a megacorporation that might or might not let us keep taking care of our patients. I'd had a good run and been able to practice pediatrics mostly without being told what to do for almost forty years. All things considered, not so bad and not such a bad time to quit.

I believed and still believe that medical records should be digitalized, and I had adopted an EMR sixteen years before they were in general use and mandatory. I had even been involved in some of the very early theoretical work on EMRs. None of my ideas came anywhere near close to being adopted. There was a bit of grandiosity back then about maybe revolutionizing medical care and becoming very rich.

Almost thirty years after all that, I was being forced to adopt an EMR system that I was sure would hurt patients and maybe put us out of business. I couldn't believe that I could be told what to do. I'd gone to medical school, had been practicing for thirty-six years, had a practice that took very good care of patients, and had an EMR system that worked well. I went around in my threadbare blue blazer, hat in hand, begging for our practice to be allowed to continue existing as an independent entity.

The preferred-provider-organization guys checked our books and the numbers worked out well enough for us to not be gobbled up. I asked my son, who was good at business, where I could buy a good but hopefully less-than-thousand-dollar suit.

I started staying up late at night doing math, then writing my friends who understood economics to check my work, and then doing more math. My calculations proved beyond a shadow of doubt that the multibillion-dollar EMR system we were being forced to adopt was going to hurt patients. The original EMR I had bought cost about two thousand dollars. As someone who grew up on Cape Cod, I notice these things.

I was going to share the math with the group of pediatricians

I was part of. They would be convinced and share it with others. Once the chain reaction started, no one would be able to stop it.

I told my practice administrator and bookkeeper to stop paying any of the bills from the EMR vendor. My practice administrator, bookkeeper, and wife were concerned. I explained that if the EMR people complained we could always pay them later and that if other practices and hospitals put off paying their EMR bills and we all did it together, the EMR folks would have to negotiate with us as a unit and change the GDMF system to one that worked. My practice administrator, bookkeeper, and wife were not reassured. I couldn't stop doing math.

If we and other practices didn't pay our EMR bills, we would drive evil people out of business. I'd be able to give everyone in my office a raise, put my grandchildren through college, build an addition on the house with a really good sound system, and buy lots of musical instruments, including a pedal steel guitar, a xylophone, and electric mandolin.

Suddenly, there was crushing chest pain and my wife and I were on our way to MGH, where it was established that my heart was fine and that a psychiatric hospital would be the best place for me.

There's a big difference between being crazy and being wrong. My math about what the new electronic medical record was going to do to medical care was, in fact, correct.

Polio 1955

As soon as a polio vaccine was available, circa 1955, my whole elementary school and many other schools lined up in the gym to get their shots. My piano teacher died from polio. A close friend spent weeks in the hospital, then had braces on his legs for years and still has a partially withered, painful leg. There used to be whole hospitals that did nothing but care for people with polio. The vaccine was free. The direct economic benefits of getting rid of polio amounted to billions upon billions—now trillions—of dollars that we now get to put to other uses.

In terms of having a positive effect on public and personal health, nothing comes close to vaccines. So why do I and so many other doctors have to spend time convincing people that vaccines are safe? It's at least partly our fault. We're the ones who went to medical school. We're supposed to be the grown-ups in this picture. Parents who are reluctant to get their children immunized are 100 percent good parents and 100 percent convinced that vaccines might hurt their child. Young parents don't come up with this stuff on their own. They are bombarded by well-meaning friends, family, and the internet. They are exhausted and overwhelmed, trying to figure out how to be parents, how to protect their child from harm. Someone coming at their baby with needles seems a more immediate threat than whooping cough.

My personal approach, which may or may not be the right one, is to not argue much because arguing often seems to do harm and just hardens the vaccine objector's position. I don't kick kids or families out of the practice. If we refused to take care of children whose parents harbored nutty or unscientific ideas, we wouldn't have much to do.

More than a few times, I've asked parents who want to talk more about vaccines and autism, "Can we please talk about something else and maybe come back to immunizations some other time?"

If I had my way, I'd make all vaccines free again, line everyone up in the gym, and put school nurses, not doctors, in charge. There's nothing about going to medical school that makes doctors qualified to give vaccines. School nurses take less crap than we do: a lot less crap.

The anti-vaccine fervor is thankfully calming down. It's sort of like a swallowed pig working its way down and out of a python—an epidemic that's burning itself out. It would help our cause and allay people's paranoid thinking if the pharmaceutical industry priced vaccines and other products more reasonably. It's not as if

I can honestly tell people that the pharmaceutical industry would never put people's health at risk to make money.

"Yes. That's all true. But your children are still better off immunized than not."

Whenever there are big profits being made, mission—the greatest good for the greatest number—suffers.

Who, exactly, are we working for?

Medical Education

A medical education is an awesome and solemn opportunity. It's almost like magic to go from applying to medical school to actually being able to change the trajectory of a human life for the better. And I felt that awesome and solemn process made me part of something much bigger than myself. It was not just another business opportunity or job.

Medical students can and do perform life-saving procedures, like putting in chest tubes, doing CPR, and bringing limp, blue babies back to life with a bag and mask and a little oxygen, but they always do so backed up by junior and senior residents who will make sure the patient doesn't die if the student screws up.

Senior pediatric residents are often sent out alone or with a nurse to stabilize and transport critically ill patients back to their home hospitals. Three years earlier these same senior residents were clueless medical students in white coats apologizing for their presence and trying not to look bewildered.

Everyone who applies to medical school does so with visions in their head of saving life and limb or of being part of a larger effort to make life better. I thought it would be relatively easy to acquire knowledge and skills that would make doing "good" almost automatic.

Unless you're a trauma surgeon in a busy ER, life is less dramatic once residency is over. Two of my patients claim I saved their lives without it being remotely true.

"Reporting for duty, sir. Send me wherever I can be of most use, sir. I'm joining up to be in the army that's on the side of angels."

There was an earnest, simple beauty to it.

Mine is the last generation to experience a time when it was still possible for doctors to be their own bosses. You could put your name on a sign and open up your own practice. You were in charge of what you did and how you did it. There was frontier justice; if you were a lousy doctor, people would stop coming to see you and you'd have to do something else for a living. There were no for-profit entities between you and your patients. It was vanishingly rare for families to go bankrupt because of medical bills. It used to be much easier to be a doctor and to get to see one.

There is no one alive who is not a direct descendent, however far back, of someone who made an important contribution to science and medicine. Who would think of withholding medications from Pasteur's seventeenth cousin once removed or Hippocrates's great-great-granddaughter to the nth power?

The public had come to trust scientific medical care because it worked and was honest. Science was not promoted or advertised or money hungry. It was not snake oil. Science works whether or not you believe in it. If science and medical care are good things, we should be careful to not let them become too scarce. If doctors were in charge, there would be a lot more care for a lot less money.

Forty years ago virtually everyone applying to medical school was idealistic and optimistic. There was a tree just to the right of Countway Library at Harvard Medical School that had been grown from a cutting from the exact same platane tree under which Hippocrates had taught his pupils the art of medicine in ancient Greece. The original is said to be the largest platane tree in Europe. What's changed over the past forty years is how expensive medical care is and how little doctors have to say about what goes on. The tree is the same.

Plastic Surgery

> "There are two kinds of operations:
> safe and foolish."
> FRANK HOLMES, M.D.

I was amazed by how much they let me do as a medical student. I'm sure there are people who would be horrified by it, but I still think having a medical student backed up by a resident backed up by a more experienced attending physician is a very safe way to care for patients; maybe even safer than having everything done by senior physicians. There's something about having medical students around that makes residents and senior physicians want to do well.

Frank Holmes, my surgical senior resident when I was a third-year medical student, taught me how to put in a chest tube to evacuate the air from a ruptured lung. Putting in a chest tube is often a life-saving procedure, especially when it's done to treat a tension pneumothorax.

A young man, about my age, cracked three ribs in a car wreck on a Saturday night near Lesley University, less than a quarter mile from the hospital. He was getting more and more out of breath because the jagged edge of one of the broken ribs had slashed his lungs. Frank Holmes would have put in the chest tube in a minute or less if I panicked or otherwise screwed it up. The patient looked at me as I inserted the tube that let out the air that was crushing his lungs and heart. When his lung ruptured, the cut part became a one-way valve that let in air when he inhaled but didn't let air out when he exhaled. Trying to breathe made things worse. The trapped air took up more and more space and was compressing his heart and lungs.

Lay the patient knee to chest with the side of the pneumo-thorax (the free air in the chest) facing up. Imagine the anterior axillary line, a line that goes from the forward-most part of the armpit down to the forward-most part of the hip. Find the top of the rib and inject local anesthetic. Make an incision just below the top of the rib. Make the incision long enough and deep enough but not too long or too deep. Take a Kelly clamp, put the tip into the incision, creep up to the top of the rib and push it through the chest wall hard enough to get into the chest cavity without hitting the lung or an artery of a major nerve and making things worse.

There is a lovely feeling, almost a soft sighing sound, when the tip of the Kelly clamp pops through the chest wall into the pleural space that surrounds the lungs. The one-way, ever-bigger balloon that has been compressing the patient's lungs and heart escapes, and the patient can breathe again. I let my own breath out as well—I'd been holding it in this whole time without realizing it. Follow the same path with a sterile chest tube over the Kelly clamp. Hook the tube up to a vacuum seal. Watch it bubble.

It felt as if it took me forever to insert the tube while the utterly calm Frank Holmes watched and walked me through it. On another occasion he let me take out an appendix—I did everything except sew things up inside. I loved surgery, especially plastic surgery. I was playing dress up—eating, sleeping, and rounding with the real doctors, taking care of real patients. Part of me wanted to be every kind of doctor, but I liked pediatrics and pediatricians best. Still, I would have maybe been good at correcting birth defects and taking care of children with major burns.

Surgeons were different, especially to a recent hippie. Frank Holmes had soft, feminine hands that could move with blinding speed. I'm sure he heard the thing about two kinds of operations, "one being safe and the other being foolish," from someone else; the point being that you don't want cowboys who make it up as they go along doing your surgery.

While I was in medical school, my first son was born. I was six years older than most of my classmates and the only one to have a baby. Everyone wanted to see him. Because I was older and had a child, I had to start making a living to support my family sooner rather than later. Had I wanted to follow through on the plastic surgery training, it would have taken an extra five years of residency, and then a fellowship would have taken me well into my mid to late thirties, which would have been a long time to be without a grown-up job and a grown-up income to pay down my grown-up debts. I had already had to borrow a fair amount of money at 18 percent interest, because it was 1976–79. But during residency I got to think about being a plastic surgeon as they let me cut sutures either too long or too short. And late at night, I put in a chest tube.

The other thing I learned in surgery is that if you're not careful, you can do a lot more harm than good, in a hurry. It takes more time to fix mistakes than it does to make them. Frank Holmes and I stayed up until dawn one night, fixing up a seriously botched operation that, because of a wrong diagnosis, had switched directions at least twice. The operation started on the left side of the stomach and ended up on the right side and behind the liver after we had to fix the inadvertently severed common bile duct. I got to do a lot of sewing that night. It was hard to remember there was a human being I had never met under all those surgical drapes. After the operation, the surgeons involved in the operation discussed who should bill for what.

Surgery, and anesthesia along with it, is where medical care has had its most dramatic and impressive changes. There are improved ways of doing old operations and entirely new operations and procedures being developed almost every day. What we do about coughs, fevers, ear infections, sore throats, and abdominal pain hasn't changed much over the past forty years, which is one of the many things I like about pediatrics.

"I always thought you'd go into psychiatry."

Not a chance in hell. I cared too much about mental health and would have gotten into too many fist fights.

God bless science and the hard-earned truths the collective "we" have discovered over six-thousand-plus years. Without the collective effort by our forebears and all their cousins and their cousins' cousins, there would be no science or medical care or surgery. I'd be blind from my detached retinas and lame from my suboptimal knees, for sure—or, more likely, dead.

A Barn in New Jersey

> "If you come to a fork in the road, take it."
> YOGI BERRA

I don't have doctors in my family, so I didn't know what to expect from medical school or being a doctor. Medical school, and whatever lay beyond, was a voyage on an uncharted sea. I have no idea how I was so sure I wanted to be a doctor, just as I still have no idea how I had been so sure that going to British Columbia to buy land and start a commune was exactly the right thing for me to be doing when I got out of college. The fact that there was a four-month psychiatric hospitalization between the two adventures might not be unrelated. I still think they were both the right things for me to be doing at the time. I take how well things have worked out as evidence that I was correct.

It's a strange kind of faith. I sometimes joke that I just wanted to be on the side of the door that opened for a change and that I thought I'd look good in a stethoscope. At the end of the day, I'm really just a religion major who wants to see what happens next.

No one would have been surprised if my story had gone badly. "Are you really Kurt Vonnegut's son? I heard you hanged yourself in a barn in New Jersey."

The scary thing is how easily that might have been true.

No one, including myself, expected me to get into medical school. I was six years older than most other applicants, had mediocre-to-poor grades as an undergraduate, and had a psychiatric history. Now I can't imagine not being a doctor or what life would be like if I'd had to do something else for a living. God bless Harvard's commitment to diversity. I was diverse for a medical school applicant in many ways.

I could write and had published some articles, which is probably why I was admitted. My eighteen-year-old straight-A-student son likes to ask, "So how did you get into Harvard?" Maybe I did it to prove to kids like him that grades aren't all that damn important.

I was recently congratulating a patient of mine on his getting into college.

"It's not Harvard," he said.

"Don't worry, Harvard isn't Harvard either."

Bone Cancer, 1979

> "When there is pain, there are no words.
> All pain is the same."
> TONI MORRISON

I was thirty-two when I started my internship at Mass General. Only a really insecure person would bother to go to Harvard Medical School and do his internship and residency at Mass General. The first patient I took care of as an intern was an eleven-year-old girl with osteogenic sarcoma who flew into Logan Airport with a note pinned to her chest that said, "TAKE ME TO MASS GENERAL. I HAVE BONE CANCER. MY MOTHER WILL COME LATER."

She was from Cape Verde. Doctors in Cape Verde and elsewhere knew that orthopedists at MGH had a special expertise and interest in bone cancer. They had pioneered and continue to pioneer ways to cut out these very aggressive cancers and save arms and legs and patients. And MGH oncologists had developed better and better chemotherapy protocols.

1

✦ ✦ ✦

Someone from the airline put her in a cab. The cab driver knew he'd be paid at the end of the ride. Mass General knew what to do, and amazingly enough, I, as a newly minted M.D., a pediatric intern, and the patient's admitting physician, sort of knew what to do, too. I could always ask for help.

Anna Maria spoke no English and had no insurance; nothing but a nine-by-twelve manila envelope with x-rays showing a big ugly osteogenic sarcoma of her partly eaten-away right distal femur, which would eventually kill her, and a chest x-ray showing at least thirty quarter-inch spheres of the cancer, which had spread to her lungs. There were doubtless hundreds more we couldn't see. Once you see more than one or two you know the game is pretty much over. She was a quiet, calm, unafraid girl.

Generations of patients, doctors, and scientists, some from Cape Verde, some from Boston, had carefully done the hard work of figuring out what could and what couldn't be done about osteo-genic sarcoma. That knowledge was like a flower fed by deep roots. Detailed knowledge about specific cancers and how to treat them is a very recent development.

Anna Maria was cared for on the fourth floor of Vin-cent-Burnham, an aging, moldy, crumbling, outdated beauty whose elevators didn't work well. We ran the stairs when we had to and sometimes we ran them just for fun, to race the elevators. It was built in 1947, the year I was born. It looked more like a hotel that rented rooms by the hour than it did a hospital. They were always about to demolish it and give pediatrics a shiny new home, but pediatrics was low on the totem pole. Small patients equals small bills and small salaries, but without us they couldn't call themselves a "general" hospital. That's what our chief of service actually told us when anyone mentioned the condition of the Vincent-Burnham building. Exterminators had to be called in on a regular basis.

The procedure room where we did spinal taps, started IVs, and performed difficult blood draws doubled as a linen closet. There were mops in the corner. It was where the surgeons put in Anna Maria's central line, an intravenous catheter threaded up close to her heart, through which she would get small doses of palliative chemotherapy and nutrition. She had no interest in food. There was a Portuguese translator, but Anna Maria never complained about anything, not even the subclavian central line for which she was mildly sedated. I learned to be comfortable with many hairy things, but sticking big needles into a child's chest, right under their collar bone, so close to their lungs and major blood vessels, wasn't one of them. Sometimes even an experienced surgeon would accidentally nick a lung, causing air to leak from the lungs into the surrounding space, my old friend pneumothorax. Fortunately this didn't happen to Anna Maria.

Anna Maria received the same world's-best care that any other patient with osteogenic sarcoma would have received at MGH. Oncologists and orthopedists learned many things from her. I got to learn how to take care of patients.

There was nothing we could have done to extend Anna Maria's life. Advanced osteogenic sarcoma has its own course and momentum, but within that course and in spite of that momentum there were opportunities to make a difference.

"Care now because it's the right thing to do. Don't just do something—stand there and pay attention. If you listen, the patient will tell you what's wrong. The attention you pay is ninety percent of the care. Besides, you don't know much yet."

I had great teachers and was part of something bigger than myself.

✦   ✦   ✦

There were no case managers, no co-pays, no deductibles, no life-time limits. The hospital bed that cost $100 per day in 1979 costs $4,000 per day today. If you're "giving away" beds to kids with bone cancer, it's easier to give away $100 than $4,000. The fact that doctors and hospitals could give away care and services back then is part of why people trusted them. When I first went into practice, my overhead per visit was approximately six dollars. If someone couldn't pay, it was no big deal. We certainly weren't going to chase them for six dollars.

Many of my teachers were not particularly sympathetic about how long and hard we worked. "The only thing wrong with working every other night is that you miss half the cases," said a beloved surgeon. I hoped and believed he was kidding, but maybe he wasn't.

Anna Maria died peacefully with her mother and aunt holding her hands. They had a room at a motel across the street. I don't know who paid for it, but her mother and aunt mostly stayed with Anna Maria, sleeping in recliner chairs or on the floor. When she died, the head of pediatric anesthesia and I were in the room in case we were needed.

At that time, we were kings of our own castles. We gave away care because it was the right thing to do. Not taking care of Anna Maria would have been an ugly thing. Whatever burnout is, there was a lot less of it back then. The brand-new glass-and-steel towers they have today are nice. Vincent-Burnham, now torn down, was definitely a pit, but it was a pit we were in charge of.

Once upon a time, it was easy for doctors and hospitals to give away care. Taking care of sick people without first verifying their insurance status is how American medical research and medical care came to be the best in the world. The cure for burnout is, quite simply, to put doctors and nurses back in charge of patient care. The side effect of such an operation would be care that is more affordable, more accessible, and more effective.

There was very little unnecessary care back then. There's a lot of it now.

NICU

Pediatric interns and residents spend a lot of time in the neonatal intensive care unit (NICU). MGH's NICU was the first
place to put preemies on ventilators. Doctors saved a lot of lives
and taught others how to do the same. Expertise radiated from
centers of excellence. Unlike most other hospitals, MGH had
no neonatal intensive care unit "fellow" between us and senior
staff, so we got more direct teaching from senior attending and
got to do most of the procedures and other work ourselves.
The day-to-day care of these fragile, tiny babies was up to us,
reinforced by senior faculty who had been doing this for years.
Combat-hardened NICU nurses jealously protected the babies
and kept us from screwing up. And they taught us stuff and pre-
tended that we were in charge. I never got over my amazement
that complete human beings could be so small. And it was even

more amazing that I, in a few quick years, came to be unafraid of them.

Our NICU was like a rundown bowling alley but smaller, with babies in their little plexiglass worlds on both sides of the alley. There was barely enough room for one regular person or two thin ones to pass between. Working in not-so-upscale surroundings made what we did somehow even better. It certainly wasn't state-of-the-art equipment that made us good.

There was a family room where the families of patients in the pediatric intensive care unit (PICU) and the NICU could hang out. One Christmas Eve when I was covering the units, I walked by the family room and saw all these very different parents playing charades. How beautiful is that?

Now each patient has their own nurse and their own room in a glass-and-steel tower, with an extra bed for parents to spend the night. It's not the same. It's better.

Residents were necessary, respected, and expected to improvise. The ICUs, the wards, the pediatric ER couldn't have survived without us. We were not assembly-line workers. Clinical knowledge and good care were intimate and organic. They spread from the ground up and out. They were not imposed from above. We had a lot to be proud of. We were always trying to do better.

Not very many people know how to put in chest tubes or tie surgical knots to hold them in place. There was no burnout. Depression, anxiety, addiction, yes, but no burnout. Burnout is different. It's about being forced to do things that don't help patients.

A doctor sees things and does things that can't be unseen or undone—gunshot wounds to the heart, third-degree burns that cover 90-plus percent of a body, callous doctors, compassionate doctors, drowned children, overdose, overdose, overdose, car wrecks up close and personal, victims of cardiac arrest rushed in by ambulance, who almost never do well, especially when trauma surgeons open the chest and massage the heart, but not zero, but not zero, but not zero . . .

I'll probably never have to put in a chest tube again, but I could if I had to. At seventy-three, I for sure won't be starting IVs in one-pound babies.

As an intern and junior resident, I had to put tiny little chest tubes into tiny little babies. I never liked waking up the senior resident. I did two chest tubes in one night. Most of our preemies, some of whom weighed two pounds or less, were on ventilators trying to push enough oxygen through their not-ready-to-be-born-yet lungs to keep them alive until the lungs could catch up. Both ventilator pressure and oxygen damaged lungs, making them stiff and prone to air leaks. It was a race between immature lungs and the side effects of what we were doing to save lives. So there I was at three a.m., putting tiny chest tubes with tiny little clamps into tiny little babies, who would have almost fit in my pocket. It was somehow normal. Humans can get used to anything.

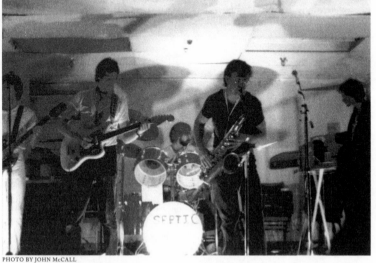

Septic Shock

> "It's only rock and roll but I like it, like it, yes, I do."
> ROLLING STONES

As interns and residents, we somehow found time to form a rock-and-roll band called Septic Shock. We were "THE WORLD'S BEST ALL-DOCTOR ROCK-AND-ROLL BAND FROM MGH." No one argued with this claim. We played, mostly for free, at parties paid for by pharmaceutical companies. They bought the beer and wine. There didn't seem to be anything wrong with it. It was 1979.

We had a few paying jobs at private parties. We were actually good. I played saxophone and still do. I play too loud and use too many notes until I get the hang of a song. They even let me sing one song—"I'm going to wait for the midnight hour. That's when my love comes tumbling down." The vocal range was three to four notes.

"Imagine how good we would be if we practiced."

✦   ✦   ✦

In the early eighties, at the end of my residency, Congress decided to open up medical care to for-profit corporations. The wisdom and efficiency of market forces would control costs and bring order and the appreciation of the insurance and pharmaceutical industries. I wish, you wish, we all wish.

It makes no more sense to privatize medical care the way we have than it does to privatize fire departments and allow them to sell variable degrees of coverage with co-payments and deductibles. They probably wouldn't cover some cities at all—like, say, Baltimore. Why should my taxes pay for your fire? Corporations got to buy what once belonged to everyone and rent it back to us one patient at a time.

While Congress was greenlighting for-profit health insurance and giving away drug patents to the pharmaceutical industry, thus relieving them of the need to do research, I went from being an ordinary guy to one who could be in charge of ICUs and pediatric emergency rooms and put chest tubes in one-pound babies. And I could and did start IVs half asleep.

My favorite scene in the movie *Butch Cassidy and the Sundance Kid* comes when Sundance admits that he doesn't want to jump from the cliff into the river, because he doesn't know how to swim.

"Are you crazy?" says Butch. "The fall will probably kill you."

As scary as it might seem to question the powers that be, we have no real choice. We have to hold hands with our patients and jump.

Before HIV had a name

> "Innocence is a kind of insanity."
> GRAHAM GREENE

Cambridge City Hospital ER, 1980.

I was a junior resident.

A year before HIV (human immunodeficiency virus) had a name, an eleven-month-old Haitian girl who had been sick with fevers and coughs and had stopped eating was brought into Cambridge City Hospital—just another sick kid. I'm not even sure why we decided to do a spinal tap. Maybe her soft spot (fontanel) was bulging slightly.

The Haitian child was not acutely ill or even very sick. In a million years I wouldn't have guessed she had tuberculosis of the brain and spinal cord. I'm not even sure I knew such a thing existed. Tuberculosis was something you read about in Russian novels.

Cambridge City Hospital was an appendage of Harvard and MGH but also a community hospital that served Cambridge's substantial Haitian, Portuguese, and other immigrant communities. Anything and everything came through the CCH emergency room. It was the wild, wild West compared to MGH, which in comparison was a well-ordered, quiet library.

One medical student, one intern, one junior resident, and a senior resident were in charge of inpatients, the ER, the delivery room, and the nursery. "We're very busy," I explained to interns. "But you will learn a lot and figure out what kind of a doctor you want to be."

Two years later, we figured out that HIV was the only way the thin, feverish, sick but not very sick child could have contracted tuberculous meningitis. She had to have been born with HIV from a mother with HIV, but it was 1979 and no one knew HIV existed.

It wasn't until 1981 that AIDS was recognized as a syndrome and everyone started wearing gloves. One of the risk factors for the infection was being Haitian. Ten million people with no money crammed into a very small space is an infectious-disease paradise.

HIV got a foothold in Haiti because, like tuberculosis, HIV has become a chronic infection mostly of poor people. Its effect on the middle and upper classes is just the tip of a very big iceberg, the base of which is called Poverty.

There's a huge reservoir of HIV, tuberculosis, hepatitis A, B, and C, along with untreated mental illness and addiction living under our bridges in our homeless population. Germs and diseases have a lousy record of staying put, especially when healthcare is an expensive, artificially scarce commodity.

We reported her as a case of tuberculosis to the health department and moved on. Just another Cambridge City Hospital oddball case.

Doctor Dan

Doctor Dan was a very, very good doctor and an even better teacher. Several years ago his big heart gave out. Losing Doctor Dan made the world a less interesting, less welcoming, and lonelier place.

Dan was the pediatric emergency room attending physician for one evening a week when I was an intern. Once or twice a year he also was the ward attending on the inpatient service. After residency, I followed in Dan's footsteps in the emergency room and on the inpatient service, because it was a good thing to do and because I wanted to be like Dan. I tried as best I could to mimic his intense singleness of purpose with patients and their problems. I think we were paid fifteen dollars per hour to teach and help out in the ER.

Almost all the patients we saw in the ER could have been taken care of much more quickly and less expensively in either of our pediatric offices or in any other of the two dozen or so local office-based pediatric practices. Doctor Dan, as an ER and ward attending, taught me throughout my residency how to take care of patients. He had an almost magical way of getting to the heart of what was wrong. He didn't order many lab tests and referred to ordering "routine" tests as "trolling the patient through the lab to see if anything bit." "Routine blood tests are routinely worthless," he said.

I pinned up a note on the ER bulletin board offering a hundred-dollar reward if anyone could show me a case where a CBC (complete blood count), the most commonly ordered blood test, told the resident something they didn't already know. Dan approved of my note, and his approval was worth way more than a hundred dollars. Some cases came close, but the reward went unclaimed until I took it down several years later.

Doctor Dan rode a bike everywhere he went and wore a beanie with a propeller on top that might have been trying to pass for a yarmulke. He often wore shorts long after everyone else had accepted that shorts weather had come and gone. It's a tribute to how good a doctor Dan was that no one seemed to notice his outfit. Patients, parents, students, nurses, lab techs, and even security guys didn't bat an eye. His intense attention to the task at hand rendered his appearance irrelevant.

Because he was a master clinician, and because of how accessible and trusted he and his office were, he saved insurers hundreds of thousands, if not millions, of dollars in ER visits and consultations. Even people who didn't know Dan trusted him. How could you not trust a guy wearing shorts and a propeller beanie in November in Boston?

✦ ✦ ✦

I think Dan thought the world would cut him some slack if he worked hard at being a really good pediatrician. Unfortunately for Dan and his patients and the rest of us, the contracts we all had to sign with the insurers included language about their being able to review our medical records and seek redress if our records didn't meet their standards. Because Dan was busy focusing on his patients and what he could do for them, he had a lot of notes that read:

"Fever, ST, inj P, TC+ Strep Throat—Amox."

Translation: Fever, sore throat, injected (bright red) pharynx, throat culture positive, strep throat—amoxicillin.

Lots of pediatricians, including myself, wrote similar or even more abbreviated notes back when we were in charge. In terms of taking good care of patients, such a note is more than adequate. But a contract is a contract, and when the insurers reviewed Dan's records, they sought redress to the tune of approximately $20K in damages. In spite of sworn statements from myself and other pediatricians that Dan's notes met community standards, Dan had to pay the insurers $12K. The idea that a good doctor, who was taking good care of patients, keeping them out of emergency rooms and off medications they didn't need, was being judged by people who never went to medical school was chilling.

Back then, there were more than twice as many independent community pediatric practices as there are now. We talked with each other and helped each other out frequently. The net effect of insurers taking control and judging providers is that half our hospitals, especially the rural hospitals and 80 percent of independent doctors, have been put out of business, and what Dan and I used to do for twenty dollars now costs two hundred dollars.

Shortly after his records were reviewed, my records were reviewed and I was found to be inadequate in terms of legibility, dating, and a few other things. There were no damages claimed. We hired a new receptionist to review our records and make sure they met the insurer standards. Overhead went up, as it always did when insurers thought up a new way to monitor physician behavior. When they monitored hospital behavior, overhead went up even more.

Doctor Dan's real job, what he did best, what he learned in medical school and residency and afterward, was how to not waste his patient's time. The idea that some insurance dweeb could judge Dan, tell him what to do, and make him pay $12,000 boggles the mind.

We weren't taught how to be told what to do, nor did we go through four years of medical school and three years of residency to be mindless drones. Having gone to medical school meant something. We practiced cost-effective care because it was the right thing to do and protected our patients from ineffective care. We didn't need carrots and sticks any more than our patients needed co-payments or deductibles.

I could never pull off wearing a beanie or shorts in December, but I do think about my clothes. I tried cowboy boots and Western shirts for a while but wasn't quite comfortable. There was no way to imitate him except to be myself, have fun, and care deeply about patients.

Dan's best public performance was a beauty. He wasn't shy. Once we were at a staff meeting in a large auditorium at Children's Hospital Medical Center. The chief of staff was explaining that specialists and hospitalists would be the only ones admitting and taking care of patients—not primary care doctors like Dan. Among other things there was a fair amount of money involved.

Dan raised and waved his hand for a while. When he was finally acknowledged by the moderator, he said, "Can Doctor Nxxx come down and kiss me?"

"Why would you want Doctor Nxxx to kiss you?"

"My mother told me that if I was about to be F'd, I should be kissed first."

The idea of not letting primary care pediatricians admit and oversee the care of their patients was dropped and remains dropped forty-plus years later.

Independent community pediatrics was truly the most cost-efficient way to do things, but over the past thirty-five years our office overhead has gone from 27 percent to 56 percent, or from roughly six dollars to ninety dollars per visit. Over half our overhead comes directly or indirectly from the arbitrary demands of health insurers. The effect of overhead and debt is that doctors and hospitals are utterly and completely dependent on insurers, whose payments make up 90-plus percent of our income. When insurers say, "Jump," doctors and hospitals say, "How high?"

I could still treat ear infections and sore throats for way less than fifty dollars if insurers would let me. Dan could too if he were still here.

The Plan

> "Profits, like sausages . . . are esteemed most by those who know least about what goes into them."
> ALVIN TOFFLER

Never in the forty-plus years that I've been directly or indirectly involved in negotiations with health maintenance organizations (HMOs) or other insurers has the quality of care been important to them. Low bid wins: always. In the beginning, health insurance was still about money but more about expanding access to care. Better access to better care made people want insurance. Doctors and hospitals were better paid. There was more money for medical education and research. It was truly a win-win-win for hospitals, patients, and insurers. Unfortunately, insurance has now become a way to create and manage hospital debt, doctor debt, and patient debt, more like a protection racket than a service industry.

✦ ✦ ✦

HMOs were and are supposed to control costs by focusing on preventive care, eliminating unnecessary tests and consultations, and having salaried primary care physicians act as "gatekeepers." Halfway through my second-year residency, the first local HMO, Community Health Plan (affectionately known as The Plan), switched their contract from Children's Hospital to MGH for pediatric emergency room and inpatient care.

There was something unseemly, and at least a little wrong, about MGH and Children's, both with their long-distinguished histories, competing for The Plan's business. It was the beginning of the end of what had been a mostly friendly, collegial relationship between hospitals. PPO (preferred provider organizations, entities that negotiate contracts between doctors and insurers) contracting also created and aggravated tensions between rural and urban medical care, primary care and specialists, this specialty versus that specialty. As soon as doctors and hospitals started competing to provide medical services for the lowest price, we were all played off each other and collegial niceties went out the window.

Forty years later, when we were forced to switch our PPO contract, I described our integrated behavioral health services and other things we were proud of. "That's all well and good, Doctor Vonnegut, but if the dollars work, nothing else matters."

"Good to know."

A few years after they came into existence, quite a few plan members were unhappy with The Plan. Patients were being denied services they felt they needed, and they felt they weren't being given enough time and attention. The Plan started providing mandatory midday and after-work training sessions for doctors about how to recognize and address patient satisfaction issues.

There are several things wrong with the assumptions that underlie how HMOs are supposed to work. Overall the amount of unnecessary care American physicians and hospitals provide is higher than it should be. Getting rid of a little or a lot of unnecessary care would be good for everyone's health, but the amount of money to be saved is negligible, especially when you're dealing with well-trained doctors. Part of our education and training was about how to minimize unnecessary care. The HMO model has not improved our performance even a little.

Audits of physicians by insurers cost patients millions upon millions of dollars. Whether or not the doctors did anything "wrong" is a minor detail. Lowering premiums, increasing employee compensation, or increasing access to care didn't work business-wise.

The belief that the inefficiencies of medical care can be easily rectified and that whoever does the rectifying should get to keep the money is a big part of why medical care is so expensive. There is no reason to believe that HMOs or any component of HMO care has in any way, shape, or form lowered the cost of medical care or improved its quality. And why was The Plan in charge of saying what was and was not unnecessary, and why wasn't this a conflict of interest?

As part of our contract with The Plan, the senior resident in the ER served as The Plan's night-call triage. Our senior resident would talk to the parent and assess whether the patient should come in and be evaluated or whether it could wait until the morning. We had nothing to gain or lose by having them come in or stay home. We were going to be hanging out in the ER anyway; another patient wasn't going to make much difference except to The Plan.

Even though The Plan was not very old at that point, there were already quite a few families with children with serious medical problems who felt they had to advocate for their children to get what they needed. These families assumed that we would "side with" The Plan and were pleasantly surprised when we agreed with them that their children needed XYZ. That probably had something to do with why we got fired.

I remember saying to one Plan-frustrated mother, whose child had come into us for the third time for prolonged seizures, "If your child has had four seizures in a month and you're not comfortable with how he's being managed, he should be seen by a pediatric neurologist. Maybe you could say you want that written in his chart."

Minimizing unnecessary care is and has always been part of what a good doctor does. The Plan didn't do it very well. Having patients who are comfortable with and confident in the care they're getting eliminates more unnecessary care than any business plan or compensation model ever could.

After a few months, we were fired from the phone-triage job because we were "inexperienced and brought too many people in." A few months after that, we learned that The Plan would not be renewing their MGH contract: they went back to Children's. "No community. No health. No plan." We liked to believe when we were fired that it reflected well on our integrity.

Dividing hospitals and doctors into favored, better-paid groups versus other, less favorably paid groups is what has happened instead. Everything else is posturing, fluff, and window dressing.

The Plan marketed itself to young high-tech startup corporations along Route 128 with mostly young, healthy employees and young, healthy families. Their per-patient medical costs were predictably much lower than they would have been if The Plan had to take care of a less selected population. They stumbled on a way to not cover "preexisting conditions" without having to use that phrase.

The Plan took their considerable profits and underbid the more traditional insurers for employer-based insurance contracts. Most people, especially those who are young and employed, need very few dollars per year in medical care. The only way for traditional insurers to compete with The Plan was to find a way to cover more low-cost patients and fewer high-cost patients. The net effect of cherry picking is that the cherry picker gets to keep the money and the rest of us get to carry the cost of taking care of the sick people who get dumped into the ranks of the uninsured and underinsured. We went to school to learn how to take care of people and now we are paid to take as little care of people as possible.

HMO executives and health insurance CEOs are now compensated in the $20–50 million per year range. There has long been a strong conviction among for-profit healthcare entities that if they're making money, they must be making healthcare better.

In 1983 an insurer introduced the idea of co-payments. In the beginning they were three dollars per visit and a minor annoyance.

"Why bother to care about three dollars?" So we didn't.

Ebola

Fever, nausea vomiting, weakness, diarrhea, internal bleeding, external bleeding, liver, kidney, and heart failure, dead in about a day. Ebola is as quick as HIV is slow, and it kills anyone who touches you. Wow.

We're spending a lot of money to keep it in Africa, but Ebola has made it through customs a few times. Thus far it has not established a beachhead. People suspected of having Ebola are seen promptly; they don't have to verify insurance, pay co-pays, or sign stuff. It's a lot like how we used to take care of everyone.

Ebola catches the eye. In the early days of the AIDS epidemic, ER docs and surgeons were afraid to take splinters out of people who might have AIDS. Rather than grab the splinter with a Kelly clamp and pull, they'd have a conference and draw straws. Now we have Ebola. Ebola reminds me of horror movies like *The Blob*, *Mars Attacks!*, and *The Brain Eaters*. It could get us all. We have to work together. Ebola is a horror movie. COVID-19 is a different horror movie.

When you add it all up and divide by time, most of the differences between AIDS, Ebola, diabetes, tuberculosis, and mental illness go away. They hurt people, cost boatloads of money, are mostly diseases of poverty, and spread from the poor to the less poor.

There are more similarities than dissimilarities between taking good care of patients with Ebola and taking good care of patients with diabetes. The job of science is exactly the same: figure out what's true and what's not true and what can be done to help.

Ebola got a lot of notice without actually having to kill very many people. While we're worrying about Ebola we should not forget to worry about six-hour ER waits, rising co-payments and deductibles, burnt-out doctors, and overworked nurses.

Mental illness, diabetes, drug addiction, and hepatitis are also "contagious," devastating, and hard to treat. Such illnesses, treatable but untreated, are unlikely to stay put in one community. There are many plagues.

The best place to treat any medical problem is where it is. The most cost-effective time to treat an illness is now. Africa is closer than we think.

Hamburger Helper

Nurse practitioners (NPs) and physician assistants are called "physician extenders." Innovation that's all about money and hardly, if at all, about healthcare is dishonest. That NPs are often good clinicians is a lucky break. Doctors who had questions about expanding the role of NPs were dismissed as money-grubbing, obstructionist cranks. To the best of my knowledge, there were no clinical studies or pilot programs, and no one ever mentioned the billions of dollars that would fall into the lap of the insurance industry.

Our NPs are absolutely wonderful. We couldn't live without them. They are excellent clinicians and, as a rule, they have fewer personality disorders than physicians do, and are easier to work with. But it's hard not to resent the fact that the point of expanding NPs' responsibilities was so that insurers could pay doctors less. Insurers saved billions of dollars, none of which made it back to patient care.

The NP thing worked out very well, so why not have more care delivered by medical assistants? They can take brief histories, draw blood, run EKGs, reconcile medication lists and allergies, and administer behavioral-health inventories. Minute clinics and urgent care centers and utilization-review advisors can get insurers more bang for fewer bucks. Less money for doctors and hospitals has put many of them out of business.

Doctors and hospitals don't really have any say in how healthcare is paid for. If an insurer says there's a five-hundred-dollar co-payment for emergency room visits, that's the way it is. Doctors and hospitals go along to get along or they go out of business.

The common belief that co-payments and prior authorizations save money and are good for us is 100 percent wrong. Just like when insurers don't cover patients with preexisting conditions, the negative effects on individual and public health and the overall cost of care go up and affordable, competent care will not be there for you should you need it.

Having slightly better access to slightly better care than some people have access to doesn't make it good care.

Twenty percent of us will have a mental-health crisis at some point in our lives. Try to find a psychiatrist or inpatient bed.

Not taking care of sick people doesn't save anyone's money but insurers'.

Too many chromosomes

> "To study the phenomenon of disease without books is to sail an uncharted sea, while to study books without patients is not to go to sea at all."
>
> WILLIAM OSLER, M.D., the father of modern medicine

Adeline had trisomy 13, an extra copy of chromosome 13, otherwise known as Patau syndrome, which is so rare that most people haven't heard of it. The life expectancy of a baby born with trisomy 13 is less than six months.

For what we've spent on babies and children we knew wouldn't walk, go to school, or live very long, we could have had several new schools, three new hospitals, or a fighter jet or two. So what?

We knew from the start that Adeline was never going to walk or talk. It was amazing she saw her first birthday, let alone her sixteenth, eighteenth, or twenty-first.

When I talked to other doctors about her—for instance, when

she needed to be hospitalized or have her cataracts fixed—they thought I was making stuff up. Adeline could not exist, but she did. However rare you believe yourself to be, she was even rarer. Once you exist, it doesn't make any difference how rare you are.

When she was born, there was a parade of doctors, medical students, and nurses wanting to see this rare newborn who would probably not live long. Among other things, there was no anus. It wouldn't be fatal in the immediate future. It was a fixable surgical problem. In view of her short projected life-span, the pain and the risks of anesthesia, her multiple heart defects and other issues, what was the right thing to do?

Amid the swirl of conflicting opinions and advice were two parents, who already had four healthy children. I was an advisor who had never seen or taken care of anyone with trisomy 13.

"Parents get to say what happens," I told them. "The surgeons and all the rest of the people examining your daughter are bystanders. There's nothing wrong with them. They all want to do the right thing, but this is a big teaching hospital and there's lots of possible right things to think about. Also, none of these people have ever met someone like Adeline before and they won't ever meet an Adeline again. Your daughter has the misfortune to be an interesting patient. You are the parents."

"What would you do?" they asked.

"If she was mine, I'd do the colostomy, which can be reversed later. We can't be sure how long she'll live, and a full bowel with no outlet is going to be uncomfortable and eventually fatal. Better now than when the bowel is distended and she's older and maybe more sensitive to pain. If you decide to do it, it will probably be the last time she has to go through surgery."

The number of times I was wrong about Adeline are legion. Her parents didn't give up on me because I kept trying to get it right.

✦　✦　✦

Once upon a time there was no life, no genetic diseases, and no chromosomes to have too many of. Then there was life but still no chromosomes. If we had stuck with reproducing by splitting in half like amoebas and other single-celled organisms, there wouldn't be genetic diseases or anyone to worry about them. The diversity that makes us interesting is a direct result of sex—the mixing, sorting, and re-sorting of genetic information. It's a messy process that allows all kinds of things to happen, like ending up with too many chromosomes.

I told the family to not bother immunizing Adeline or doing much about her blindness or deafness or getting a cardiac consult for her complex congenital heart disease, because she wouldn't, couldn't, live very long. Eventually, we ended up doing all that and more.

My wife and I went to her sixteenth birthday party, complete with ice-cream cake and a pony. If you have a hard time being wrong, don't become a doctor. Or learn how to get over it.

Parading cute, unfortunate children across our TV screens to ask for money is disturbing. Taking care of such children should be a routine part of what we, as a society, do—not something we fund with bake sales or GoFundMe pleas. Once upon a time we managed to take care of such children without TV ads. I have nothing against the people who run such campaigns but regret that the practice seems to be necessary. It would be way less expensive to just take care of sick people.

You are the parent. If your child has the misfortune to be born an interesting patient, there will be specialists. There will be medical students, sweet, well-intentioned, and incredibly young. You will also have family and neighbors, some of whom have opinions and want to help.

Interesting babies are more like other babies than not. Feed the baby. Keep the baby warm. Don't let her brothers and sisters poke her in the eyes. Smile nicely and nod when relatives give you advice.

Adeline had a colostomy shortly after she was born. She also had her cataracts removed and multiple ear, nose, and throat procedures to restore her hearing, though what she saw or heard was anyone's guess. At each decision point my initial reaction was more likely to be wrong than right.

Me: "Her life expectancy is less than six months, we shouldn't bother to immunize her."

Her parents: "She's in the backyard playing with her siblings or her siblings are playing with her. She seems to be enjoying it. What about a tetanus shot?"

She ended up fully immunized.

Her parents: "Should she see a geneticist?"

Me: "Why?"

Her parents: "Should she see a cardiologist?"

Me: "Why?"

She ended up seeing both a geneticist and a cardiologist.

Parenting a chronically sick or disabled child is a full-time job. The doctor's job should be to speak when spoken to and try to not have too many opinions.

Her siblings all grew up to be wonderful people, two of whom went into healthcare. How much Adeline has to do with how her siblings turned out is anyone's guess, which is sort of the point.

She had several pneumonias in her early twenties. They were unusual, probably not infectious pneumonias. Her lungs scarred down with each pneumonia but never healed. It's not like I could look up twenty-three-year-old patients with trisomy 13 and pneumonia to help us figure out what might be going on and what to do about it. She finally seemed tired and was let go at twenty-three years old, far and away the oldest patient with trisomy 13, which wasn't the point.

Adeline and other children born with genetic diseases are what insurance companies call "high utilizers." They send us lists of our "high utilizers" as if there was something we could or should be doing about them.

If you do the math, "high utilizers" don't cost us any more than anyone else. Not taking care of them, for whatever reason, is a slippery slope at the end of which we don't take care of anyone.

When the Make-A-Wish people asked if Adeline would enjoy a trip to Disneyland, I honestly didn't know, "—but her brothers and sisters and parents could use a trip to Disney, and that's probably the best thing we can do for Adeline." She seemed to like being around and sort of playing with her siblings, which was a big part of why we did all that other stuff. I think she liked sitting on the pony at her sixteenth birthday party. She taught me more about pediatrics than anyone else.

Pediatrics

> "Parents don't make mistakes because they
> don't care, but because they care so deeply."
> T. BERRY BRAZELTON, M.D.

All parents want to be good parents. A huge part of what a pediatrician does is to help parents be the best parents they can be. Babies who don't get continuous attention and care don't live very long. Thankfully we don't have to be perfect parents; we just have to be "good enough." Feed the baby. Keep the baby warm. Change the baby's diapers. I think babies should be picked up when they cry but not everyone agrees.

Babies and people in general are incredibly resilient. Telling and hearing stories is a huge part of how and why we survive. Most of the stories we tell are about surviving horrible things. People are all helpless babies who don't last long or do well without care. Medical care has been around for as long as we've had stories. Like it or not, we are our brothers' keepers. Who else?

Most of what pediatricians get paid to treat are ear infections, sore throats, vomiting, fever, cough, diarrhea, and rashes. Brief office visits are now known by the insurance industry as 99213s. And we do well baby and well child visits, during which I usually find very little wrong with the patient. I am mostly checking with the parents, especially the mother, to make sure that they're doing OK. I've been doing these things long enough that I could treat ear infections, coughs, and fevers in my sleep, but I don't, and it's the "but I don't" that makes pediatrics an occasion worth rising to. Very few of my patients would have died if not for my care. But not zero. But not zero. But not zero.

Fever, cough, rash, runny nose, cough, vomiting, vomiting and diarrhea with or without fever and cough and rash. My baby won't eat. Why won't my baby stop crying?

I learned pathophysiology, pharmacology, and some other things in medical school, and I learned physical diagnosis and clinical logic as an intern and resident, but I've learned how to do what I do mostly from my patients, who have been and still are very patient teachers. They very much want me to get it right.

I hope the current money poisoning comes to an end, or doctors and nurses find ways around it, so we can get back to having medical care be about helping patients. It's the best job in the world; the job 99 percent of us set out to do.

Forty years ago pediatric office visits cost ten, fifteen, and twenty dollars, which just about everyone could afford, and it felt right. Then and now, patients pay for everything, but back then, "everything" cost a lot less than it does now. We pediatricians were only slightly jealous of surgeons or specialists, who made more. No one looked down on us because we made less money.

Our visits back then were mostly about minor infections. But more serious diagnoses tried to sneak through, and identifying them was like picking out needles in a haystack. We prided ourselves on not missing the needles, but what we were doing was mostly helping parents learn how to be more comfortable with their children. While we were taking care of minor infections and reassuring nervous parents, we were keeping babies and children out of hospitals and emergency rooms, off unnecessary medications, and away from quacks. We were an important, integral part of medical care. Doctors talked to each other much more back then. We used telephones and it made the world a safer place.

Our overhead was low and life was good. We weighed and measured babies ourselves and did our own vital signs and immunizations. Our community felt connected to us and trusted us. People didn't Google everything we said and refuse vaccines. When it was the right thing to do, we made house calls. When it was the right thing to do, we gave away care.

The thing I like best about being a boss is not having to have one. We take care of whoever shows up. We do not discriminate against insurance status or parental lunacy. People with imperfect parents deserve and need good care as much as or more than the ones with allegedly normal parents.

You can't be happy working in a pediatric office and saying "no" more than once or twice a week. If "no" has to be said, it should be done as a team effort. The patient comes first, second, and third. It helps to make eye contact and not be depressed, distracted, or typing while the parent or patient is talking.

I call my office the pediatric commune and sometimes ask if there's anyone who feels like giving immunizations, bringing back patients, doing a nebulizer treatment, or answering the damn phone. It's been mostly fun being in charge of an office full of people, mostly because we mostly hire people who mostly don't need me to be the boss. I try to be more like a trusted servant than a top-down leader.

We have three receptionists, four nurses, two medical assistants, five social workers, a biller, a bookkeeper, an IT guy, a practice administrator, a medical home coordinator, four doctors, five nurse practitioners, a psychopharmacologist, and a wife who checks over the numbers to make sure we have enough money and that no one is robbing us blind. Without a wife, a bookkeeper, and a practice administrator, I'd be dead in the water.

We ask people how much they want to work and what we should pay them. It's better than trying to read their minds, and they often want to be paid less than what I would have guessed. Rather than fire people, I've occasionally had to resign as their boss.

Our note to new parents:

You are the parent.

To thrive, your baby has to eat, sleep, and stay warm.

If you keep the baby with you most of the time and are holding the baby most of the time, the baby will stay warm. If it is a skinny baby, socks and a hat will help. Babies don't need the thermostat set at eighty degrees. Their hands and feet should be slightly cooler than their bellies. If they are too cold, their hands and feet will be clenched, slightly blue, and cold.

Nothing brings out the advisor in people like a new baby, especially a new healthy baby, especially a new healthy baby born to novice parents. Prior to having a child, most of us are blissfully unaware of the volumes of wisdom our friends and families have about exactly what you should and shouldn't do with a baby. For all their differences, friends, family, and would-be advisors share a key attribute: they are not the parents. They will not be doing the breastfeeding or the formula feeding, the getting up with, the letting cry, the not letting cry, the swaddling, the not swaddling, the letting them have a pacifier, the not letting them have a pacifier, the keeping their room warm or cold, the hat or no hat, the pierced ears, the not-pierced ears. However different new parents are, you share the same very important, very recent, earth-shattering change of status: you are the parents.

Whether the baby is big or small, bottle fed or breastfed, African, European, Asian, or Native American, there are almost no exceptions to the following rules:

1. If the baby is hungry, feed the baby.
2. If the baby is asleep, let the baby sleep.
3. Listen attentively to relatives but don't do what they say.
4. Enlarging upon these rules and looking for exceptions is more trouble than it's worth.

Trust your heart. Your instincts have evolved over millions of years. You can probably trust them. If a mistake is made as a result of following your feelings it's unlikely to be a serious one and not nearly as dangerous as the mistakes we make ignoring our instincts. Babies are designed to withstand bad advice and novice mistakes, so please try to enjoy being a new parent. These days won't come again.

Babies like the color red and can't get enough of being talked to.

Parents worry a lot about things that their children turn out not to have, which is a good thing. I would rather see fifty patients with nothing much wrong than miss one who is seriously ill. Most of the patients we see during our walk-in hour or for sick visits later in the day have minor viral illnesses and symptoms that would go away on their own. This is also a good thing. Eventually, maybe, we can teach people how to not sweat the small stuff.

Some of us will never not sweat the small stuff. Welcome to the club.

Our job is to explain and make available what science knows and what it doesn't know. Science was developed by and for all of us to produce the most good for the most people. That was a scientific reality, not some liberal pie-in-the-sky pipe dream. The current conflict between the money of medical care and the mission of medical care is a major public-health issue.

In pediatrics, and most medical care, if the doctor can just shut up and listen long enough, the patient will reveal the diagnosis. Unfortunately, there's not a procedure code or template for how to shut up.

Anemia

> "The soul is healed by being with children."
> FYODOR DOSTOEVSKY

Marlow Conrad was sick a lot. At first we thought he probably had run-of-the-mill viruses and nickel-dime iron deficiency: eat-more-cheeseburgers, maybe-take-some-iron anemia. Anemia is extremely common. We test all babies for it when they're about twelve months old. It makes a difference.

But Marlow's anemia got worse. His platelets and white count went down. His bone marrow wasn't doing anything right. He had aplastic anemia, which was among the things I thought I might have when I was unexpectedly found to be seriously anemic last year. Thankfully my anemia got better before the hematologists could do anything about it. Aplastic anemia doesn't get better suddenly or even slowly. Marlow stopped growing.

Apart from transfusions to make him feel better and keep him alive, the only thing that was going to really help Marlow was a bone-marrow transplant. Marlow's four brothers all looked like carbon copies of him, but neither they nor anyone else in the family was a good enough match to be a bone-marrow donor.

Mrs. Conrad got pregnant. I remember a hematology fellow saying something about it not being right to have a baby to be a bone-marrow donor. And I thought, why the F not? Feel free to call in social work and child-protection services. It wasn't as if they would have sold the baby or put it up for adoption if the tissue typing hadn't worked out. The Conrads would have just kept trying.

The new baby was a perfect match. Nice. Once he was big enough, his bone marrow was harvested, cleaned up, made ready, put in a giant syringe, and infused into his anesthetized brother. There were no complications. The youngest brother, the much-wanted sixth son, grew up to be the biggest, strongest, handsomest brother of all.

I love routine days with routine patients, if there is such a thing as routine patients, but being close to stories like Marlow's makes the routine even better. I get a front-row seat and, every once in a while, a chance to be useful.

Brittle Bones

Before Caleb Wilson was born, his mother came to me and said the child she was carrying had osteogenesis imperfecta (OI), or imperfect bones. "Imperfect" is an understatement. The bones of babies and children with OI are as fragile as eggshells; they fracture if you so much as pick the baby up. The parents had been advised to have an abortion, but they weren't going to do that. They had two healthy children. They wanted to know what I thought. What I thought was: these are very brave people.

Even with maternal bed rest and an extra-gentle C-section and handling at birth, Caleb was born with over one hundred fractures. Caleb is the one and only child with osteogenesis imperfecta I or anyone else in my practice has ever seen or is likely to see; it's a rare condition. But if you have a one-in-a-million disease you still get 100 percent of it, not just a millionth.

Caleb's family had been paying routine premiums for their high-cost private insurance for many years. Shortly after he was born, an insurance case manager care coordinator called his father and told him about a special program for children with special needs, like Caleb. The program was MassHealth, our version of Medicaid, which would pay for the special car bed and orthopedic consults he would need.

It's a good thing that children like Caleb are covered and taken care of by Medicaid, but it's worth noting that, somewhere in the fine print, Medicaid, along with helping poor patients and their families, also acts as a safety net for the insurance industry. After taking $20,000 per year for years from the Wilsons, their private insurer got out of taking any responsibility for Caleb's care by dumping it on Medicaid. They continued to insure the rest of the family. Good work if you can get it.

Little by little by little, Caleb learned how to walk and not to shatter bones so easily in the process. When it was necessary, his father and I would gently take him out of his special portable car crib and carefully lie him on a special foam-rubber exam-table pad like the brittle egg he was.

Programs to take care of children with "prolonged illness conditions" often require letters of medical necessity to make sure patients still qualify for special beds and wheelchairs. I've actually had to write notes to an insurer that said, "Maggie still has no left leg. She continues to grow and will need a new prosthesis."

It's not uncommon now for families of children with cancer to end up bankrupt due to co-pays and other out-of-pocket expenses. Forty years ago it was punishment enough to have a child with cancer, and virtually no one went broke because of medical care.

No one fakes the need for a special car bed or an artificial leg. I have a special nurse to fill out prior authorizations to prevent steam from coming out of my ears. Monitoring and second-guessing doctors costs millions upon millions of dollars and has never saved patients a dime. Those dollars have never found their way back into patient care.

Caleb is very smart and empathetic, like lots of other chronically ill children. His legs are severely bowed from his many fractures. He gets around. My favorite image of Caleb is of him sitting on his father's shoulders like Tiny Tim in Dickens's *Christmas Carol*.

"God bless us, every one!"

Insulin

Science is supposed to change how we see the world. Prior to the discovery of insulin in the early 1920s, type 1 diabetes was a brutal, universally fatal disease. Victims, almost always children, were unable to metabolize sugar and slowly starved to death or died from dehydration. Food made their symptoms worse. The only thing that delayed death for diabetics was to eat as little as possible for as long as possible.

Doctors Frederick Banting and Charles Best, the discoverers of insulin, sold the commercial rights to the drug for four dollars. The idea was that insulin should and would be made as widely available as possible. Initially that's pretty much what happened. The pharmaceutical industry and everyone else worked hard and together to make insulin widely available and affordable. Diabetes was transformed from a death sentence to a manageable disease. Diabetics were able to live 90-plus percent normal lives and pharmaceutical manufacturers made a reasonable profit.

But over time, insulin's monopoly, jealously guarded and protected by lawyers, has allowed manufacturers to create artificial scarcity and prevent competition. Now they make an entirely unreasonable profit that goes to investors and upper management. We have, essentially, re-created diabetes and all its complications. Diabetes is now the leading cause of blindness, amputation, and kidney failure. Untreated and undertreated diabetics fill our ambulances and emergency rooms, and they eat up huge chunks of the Veterans Affairs, Medicare, and Medicaid budgets. At the outset it was unthinkable that a pharmaceutical corporation would create scarcity to increase the price of a drug. Now it's routine.

It would be nice if the pharmaceutical industry took the many billions of dollars it makes on insulin and used those dollars to support research that brings us new and better drugs. Unfortunately that's not where the money goes. Big profits attract investors and money. There's no reason to believe that the prospect of great wealth drives great discoveries. We now have dozens of blockbuster, billion-plus-dollar drugs on the way, but the net effect of these drugs is, more often than not, negative. Patients and their families are held over a barrel. Dollars that could have gone to more important research or clinical care get gobbled up.

The chance that the manufacturers of insulin don't know that they're killing people is zero, or about the same as the chance that the manufacturers of oxycontin didn't know their product was addictive. Pharmaceutical corporations freely admit that their number-one job is making money. The best way for a pharmaceutical company to make money is to do as little research as possible while jacking prices through the roof. While they claim to be doing useful research, the truth is that most of what they call "research" is devoted to prolonging monopolies on existing drugs.

Science is supposed to change things for the better. Making rich people richer doesn't make things better. Everybody has to eat but good science has always been done, mostly for curiosity, with a little bit, or more than a little bit, of ego thrown in. From ancient Greece to the Renaissance to today, useful science gets discovered when it's ready to get discovered. Had Banting and Best not isolated and identified insulin when they did, there were several other scientists hot on the trail who would have done so within a year.

Taking scientists and giving them money for the express purpose of developing blockbuster drugs is an unseemly waste of everybody's time.

During World War II, German diabetics learned how to make their own insulin. The technology is much simpler now, and high-quality home-brewed insulin could become a reality in the not-distant future. I imagine diabetic cooperatives having their own five-gallon insulin-fermentation-and-harvesting kits. Widely available cheap insulin would be a major public-health advance, equal in magnitude and scope to the current public-health disaster of artificially scarce insulin.

Science for hire isn't really science. By making everything cost so much, we are effectively un-discovering penicillin, insulin, and vaccines. We're moving away from where science and scientists want us to go.

Generations of scientists, patients, and doctors have worked very hard to create safe, effective drugs. This same science has now been weaponized against the very people scientists were trying to help.

There are renegade biochemists currently working on home-brewed insulin. They call themselves bio-hackers. Sign me up and bring it on.

Frankie

Mother: "He throws up and then seems fine. He does it at least once a week and sometimes three or four times. No fever, no diarrhea. Nothing."

"Frankie, do you feel sick or have any pain when you throw up?"

"No, not really. I think it's eggplant. It tastes slimy to me. Every time I eat eggplant I throw up. I tried to tell my mom but she didn't believe me."

Mother: "No one's allergic to eggplant and I think it happens other times, too."

"Let's run the experiment of not eating eggplant for two weeks and see what happens."

His mother reluctantly agreed to stop feeding Frankie eggplant and Frankie stopped throwing up.

Maybe someday he'll bring his kids to me.

The Worst Mother in the World

> "Sell your cleverness and buy bewilderment. Cleverness is mere opinion. Bewilderment brings intuitive knowledge."
>
> RUMI

"Am I the worst mother in the world?"

There are mothers who are so angry and indifferent to the needs of their children and so abusive to our nurses and staff that they frighten me. They are true psychopaths. It would not occur to them that they might be The Worst Mother in the World (TWMITW), nor would they care if anyone said anything to them about it. Their children seem patient and mature beyond their years. In the short run having TWMITW as your mother is nowhere near as damaging as I would have thought.

"I must be the worst mother in the world." It's usually said lightly by a mother who knows she's not so bad. However, two or three times a year a mother breaks down crying, believing that she's for real the worst mother in the world. I've never had a father worry seriously about being "the worst father in the world." Maybe the criteria for good fathering are less demanding.

"The worst mother in the world was actually here earlier and we're very glad she's gone. You're not even in the top ten. If you're serious about being TWMITW, you've got to do more than miss the symptoms of an ear infection, be late for or miss an appointment, or bring in a child with dirty feet and mismatched socks."

But when the question is serious, mothers, usually young, usually isolated, not infrequently with critical in-laws and mothers, truly believe that they are failing at the most important job in the world and the thing they most want to be good at.

If a mother-in-law, husband, sister, teacher, or stranger on the street says anything or looks askance at a mother who is herself wondering whether she's doing a good job, especially if she's sleep deprived or the baby is crying, some mothers come to believe that they are not good mothers. It's almost always very good mothers with more than one or two children who believe that they are TWMITW.

"I promise that you're not even a slightly bad mother. You need to sleep, to see some friends, and to tell whoever is making you feel this way to buzz off."

If we needed perfect mothers, the human race would have died out a long time ago. All we need are mothers who are "good enough." There are billions of years of motherhood that include enormous amounts of accumulated wisdom. It's a relatively recent phenomenon that so many mothers have babies without the physical presence, help, and comfort of their own mothers, sisters, aunts, and lifelong friends. Along with relative social isolation many mothers pay the price of not having access to the accumulated wisdom of how to mother and how to survive being a mother. A key part of that wisdom, I'm convinced, is how to tell unhelpful critics and would-be coaches to FO. A new mother apart from her herd is vulnerable like a wildebeest.

Over the years I have watched many mothers who thought they were bad mothers toughen up and tell their critics, including the inner one, to buzz off. It's our secret that once upon a time they believed themselves to be TWMITW.

When should I panic?

Not knowing when to panic and being the worst mother in the world are closely related: if you know when to panic you cannot be TWMITW, because there are other mothers who don't know when they should panic.

Reassuring people, telling them not to worry, doesn't work. Parents get tougher over time, but it doesn't help to dismiss their concerns. I sometimes ask, "Why are you dragging such a healthy-looking child into a pediatric office?" I do it only if the baby or child looks perfectly healthy. And I do it with a smile. The parent then gives me a history of symptoms and tells me what they're worried about. I then go about proving that the patient either does or doesn't have an ear infection, pneumonia, flu, Lyme disease . . .

Most minor illnesses would probably get better by themselves. We teach parents how to treat fevers, vomiting and diarrhea, coughs, and other symptoms. We also tell them the child will be well again soon but to call us again if things don't get better, especially if things get worse or there are new symptoms.

Even when patients have a more serious infection like pneumonia or a more complicated infection like Lyme disease, we can often deal with it without x-rays, specialists, or blood tests. But still the question remains, even if parents don't ask it, "What if they don't get better? When should I panic? When should I call back?"

Especially if I'm 99 percent sure the patient will get better, I try to lighten the mood: "You can call anytime. You can panic now. You're here. I'm here. I've got some extra time. Three a.m. is not a good time to panic. Especially if you're alone. If they don't get better we can do X, Y, or Z, but even if we have to do X, Y, or Z, even if they have A, B, or C, it's all compatible with a long, happy life."

"We are not going to let this go on forever."

"We will not abandon you even if you panic."

"Doctor, is everything possible being done?"

"I hope not. When doctors do everything, it's a sure sign that they don't know what's going on."

Modern surgery and effective medication have had the unfortunate side effects of making us think there's always a dramatic procedure or test to be done, a cure to be had. Most people aren't comfortable anymore with the idea of not doing something even when they know that doing something is not likely to help. The concept of when to panic didn't come up in medical school. Doctors don't know when to panic either, so we stay busy and hope for the best.

Lead Poisoning

> "Our children are our greatest treasure.
> They are our future."
> NELSON MANDELA

Lead paint is excellent paint. It covers better and lasts longer than non-lead paint, which means that, before it was banned, we used a lot of it. Lead dust and scraped paint chips are everywhere. Even though it's been illegal to use lead paint since 1978 it can still be found in many houses and apartments. It's also illegal to rent or sell an apartment or house that has lead paint to any family with young children.

Lead paint tastes good and you can chew it like gum. It's much more toxic to the developing brain than it is to the so-called mature brain. Most children with lead poisoning are children who, because of a lack of choice, live in substandard housing. The odds that slumlords who rent to families with young children don't know that they are poisoning young brains are zero.

Many years ago I was called into court to testify that one of my patients, whose family lived in substandard housing that was loaded with lead paint, had developmental delays and sky-high lead levels. It seemed like an open-and-shut case. I assumed the landlord would just say he was sorry and pay up. It didn't occur to me that the cheap-suit landlord with the cheap-suit lawyer could get away with poisoning children.

My naive self was surprised to be cross-examined about how I knew that lead poisoning in general caused harm and that lead poisoning was responsible for my patient's problems. Was I an expert on lead poisoning? And so forth.

I think I held my own but was surprised and more than a little upset when the landlord got off with a small settlement that would easily fit into his budget as a slumlord's cost of doing business.

I like stories where patients do well in spite of what I like to call "suboptimal" test results. I like to tell parents of slightly older children who have elevated lead levels about Brendan, who at age five had a very high lead level of 40 (a normal lead level is less than 3). We never figured out where the lead was coming from and it went down quickly without our doing much. Brendan went on to be valedictorian of Boston College High School. Imagine how smart he would have been without the lead poisoning.

The girl who was allergic to Christmas

> "When you have eliminated the impossible, whatever remains, however improbable, must be the truth."
>
> SHERLOCK HOLMES
> (Arthur C. Doyle, M.D.)

Every year like clockwork, just before Christmas, Jessica ended up in the hospital, where she had to be treated with large doses of steroids and continuous nebulized bronchodilators. One year she had a pneumopericardium, which most of us had never seen before. Air broke through her thick, stiff, worn-out asthmatic lungs and found its way into the sack around her heart. On x-ray her heart was outlined by a clear black halo. The air had to be removed by putting a needle very carefully into the space between her heart and the connective-tissue lining. It was one of the things that happened to Jessica that didn't seem to happen to other people, even other serious asthmatics.

Asthma is a serious chronic disease and the most common reason children end up in emergency rooms or admitted to hospitals. Children with asthma are sick and out of school much more often than other children and can have a hard time participating in sports. We have better medicines than we used to, medicines that prevent asthma attacks. Pediatricians are all over anything that helps us take better care of asthmatics.

For the past twenty-plus years there have been programs mandated by insurers that are intended to improve how doctors treat asthma. These programs require that doctors give their patients asthma action plans that have both cartoons and written descriptions of symptoms and what to do about them. We had to hand out these plans and document that we had done so or we wouldn't get paid. There's not an ounce of evidence to support the idea that asthma action plans help asthmatics or have done anything but increase the cost of having and treating asthma.

My asthma action plan was much simpler: "If you're looking for your asthma action plan to figure out what to do, you should probably call us." My asthma plan for older kids is: "If you're wheezing, tell your mother."

The parents of severe asthmatics like Jessica know what to do and when to call. They have systemic steroids in the medicine cabinet and have already started them by the time they call. There were often more than a few asthma action plans blowing around our parking lot.

In general, if a doctor or hospital cares and is already doing a good job, a quality improvement initiative (QI) like asthma action plans won't improve quality. If patients are doing poorly because they can't afford medications or get to follow-up appointments, no asthma action plan is going to keep them out of the ER.

Our practice, and most pediatric practices, take good care of asthmatics in spite of QI programs rather than because of them. If there's a pediatrician who finds these programs helpful I haven't met him or her. If there's a pediatrician doing such a lousy job with asthmatics that they find asthma QI programs helpful, they should go back to medical school and redo their residency.

Jessica was allergic to Christmas trees. It was her pulmonologist who figured it out. There was no blood test for that, but once the family started using a metal tree, Jessica no longer had to spend Christmases in the hospital.

Before implementing asthma quality improvement programs, asthma action plans, asthma control tests, etc., there should have been a modicum of critical thinking and maybe some science. Progress in how we take care of patients always has and always will come from careful science.

There are a large number of insurance-based edicts and programs that were supposed to control costs or improve quality that have ended up doing exactly the opposite; costs went up and the quality of care went down. Co-pays, deductibles, lifetime limits, prior authorizations, and dozens of other programs have given insurers more and more money and power. They cost boatloads of dollars and jack up everyone's insurance premiums.

Our asthma composite performance metric and other numbers are good, so, for now, we get paid well. Our numbers are good because of our demographics; we take care of mostly suburban families with mostly good insurance. Our good numbers mean we can afford to take care of everyone.

For now.

The girl with one eye

> "In the land of the blind, the one-eyed man is king."
> ERASMUS

Polly Martin was a baby born to a forty-year-old single woman. It's harder for older people to have a baby. It's not just the getting pregnant and carrying a pregnancy to term. It's everything.

Everything is easier when you're twenty years old and know you can probably have more babies if you want and you can stay up all night, no problem. Late-in-life babies are "buzzer beaters."

Teenagers and people in their early twenties can get pregnant, have the baby or twins, nurse them, transition to solid food, get them to sleep all night, leave them with babysitters with barely a second thought. They don't buy books about parenting or child development. They don't get upset if their baby doesn't roll over at four months or won't eat vegetables.

Polly was born with one eye. The left eye was actually there but so small it might just as well have not been.

Mostly for cosmetic reasons, it was decided to clean up the eye socket and give her a glass eye very early on. Eyes don't grow much and a baby with an eye patch begets too much concern, sympathy, and curiosity. When she was about eighteen months old, before she could talk much, Polly would wait for little old ladies to stick their face in hers to say how cute she was, let them get close, pop out her glass eye, and put it in her mouth.

Polly is a genius.

Honduras

> "Happiness is nothing more than good health and a bad memory."
> ALBERT SCHWEITZER, M.D.

Ten years out of residency I went to Honduras as part of a medical mission. One hundred thirteen people was way too many to go on a ten-day combined dental and medical mission to Honduras. We had optometrists, pharmacists, and a chiropractor, as well as assorted family, some of whom spoke Spanish and the rest of whom would be useful any way they could. With a hundred-plus people, the odds were zero that stupid, embarrassing things wouldn't happen. I knew only two of the other people on the mission, the emergency room doc who recruited me and a dentist.

Along with the chance to be of service, doctors and nurses should go to places like Haiti and Honduras to see that people who have never seen a doctor can be wonderfully healthy. I was excited about the chance to practice medicine beyond the confines of Route 128, see exotic diseases, and take care of desperately sick children. Parents wouldn't be demanding or entitled.

We had followed leaders with flags through airports and customs so we wouldn't lose anyone.

We were all volunteers, paying our own way. The medicines and medical supplies we brought were donated. Posters advertising our mission clinic were posted up and down the coast.

The first stupid, embarrassing thing I saw was one of the dentists throwing money from our bus to the throng of children who had gathered to see what might happen. The children, like schools of tiny tropical fish, attacked the coins as if the coins were bread crumbs.

The prime minister of Honduras had been on the plane that flew us down from Texas. The prime minister and leaders of the mission chatted up a storm. I assumed he was grateful that we were coming to care for the Honduran people. We thought that we would be taking care of people for free, but on the evening before the mission was to open, at what we expected would be a pro forma welcome meeting, the principal of the local school told us that patients would be charged forty lempira each, or about fifty cents, and that money would be used for much-needed improvements to the school.

All hell broke loose. Especially among the dentists who had come down several times before. They announced that they were going to head out into remote villages and take care of people for free, live in local homes, eat local food, and sleep in local hammocks. Anyone else from the mission who wanted to go with them was welcome to do so. It sounded like a great idea, but maybe I wasn't prepared to be a non-Spanish-speaking, translator-less, solo-traveling pediatrician. Job one would be explaining to people who had never seen a pediatrician before what it was I did. A dentist, pulling teeth, in a country where Coke was cheaper than water and most mouths had at least as many rotten teeth as healthy ones, needed no explanation. Just show them your special pliers and point at your mouth.

There was talk about not opening the clinic at all, but then what was the trip for? What were we going to spend the week doing? Sightseeing and buying souvenirs and throwing quarters at kids? Most of the group elected to stay in the commandeered plush resort hotel that had initially been built for the exclusive use of United Fruit employees and their families.

"If there are people too poor to pay, can we pay for them?" They gave us a roll of one hundred red tickets that we could use to get patients in without paying.

Monday, day one, there were what looked like several hundred people waiting at the gate. Security was provided by very young, probably teenaged soldiers in battle fatigues, with assault rifles slung over their shoulders. They had arrived by bike. "Maybe most of these people are here to see the dentists," I said to my hopeful self. We had six dentists who were set up on a large porch to yank teeth. There were lots of people with lots of rotten, presumably painful teeth. Otherwise, why would you stand in a line watching blood and teeth spit and spew out of other people's mouths while waiting your turn? A local health official during the meeting the night before had asked the dentists to please refrain from pulling more than three teeth per patient because of how many patients had ended up dangerously anemic from a previous dental mission.

At the end of the clinic day, the people still waiting in line were given numbers to save their place. There were special buses from nearby cities to bring people to our clinic. It amazed me how many people were willing to stand quietly and patiently in line for a chance to see us.

The cinderblock, barebones school had no electricity. We had to recharge our otoscopes and ophthalmoscopes back at the resort. The school had a courtyard where the kids did gymnastics, played soccer with a crumpled-paper-and-duct-tape ball, and watched adults get their teeth pulled.

I had a trio of twelve-year-old-girl translators from the local parochial school. They wore their matching school outfits. The translations were mostly fluent but they would occasionally huddle to come up with a committee decision.

A few times I wished I could snap my fingers and have a specialist appear, twice I wished I could get a chest x-ray, but never once did I wish someone had better insurance. There was an emaciated teenager dying slowly of end-stage congestive heart failure. There was a two-year-old with congenital hypothyroidism who hadn't grown at all. I was assured that, yes, these patients, even if there wasn't much that could be done to help them, would be seen by specialists in Tegucigalpa, the capital city of Honduras—". . . definitely, of course, no problem, doctor."

My translators had range. An agitated young man, staggering from either exhaustion or intoxication, was disrupting the adult side of our makeshift clinic. He was trying to stop drinking and couldn't take it anymore. He needed to sleep. He needed help. My trio of angel translators and a significant number of other Hondurans approached him, congratulating him on asking for help. You're not alone. Don't drink, go to meetings, ask for help. The whole clinic was nodding empathetically. He calmed down. People seemed to be taking care of him. I went back to my pediatric station to reassure a mother that her four-year-old was in remarkably good health in spite of refusing to eat vegetables.

At first there didn't seem to be that many children in line but by the end of the week a nurse practitioner I was allegedly supervising and I had seen roughly eight hundred children. Eight hundred times fifty cents equals four hundred dollars. That money plus whatever the adult doctors, optometrists, dentists, and chiropractor brought in buys a lot of school improvement in Honduras.

The chiropractor set up his table in an open area where waiting patients and those who had been seen could watch. He was far and away the most popular practitioner. He was tall and handsome, and he had flair.

I was surprised by how run of the mill most of the problems were. Like back home, parents mostly just wanted to be reassured that their children didn't have anything dreadful. Dreadful versus not dreadful is what I do best.

The different and great thing about practicing medicine in Honduras, for all the things that went wrong and all the things that could have been done better, was that doctors and nurses were actually in charge. The fact that we had gone to nursing school and medical school mattered.

At the end of the week, I was able to take a few hours off to visit an orphanage where I saw some patients who were in need of medical attention. I was actually able to be useful. I taught the staff in the orphanage how to get rid of warts and promised to send them urine detectors (Wet Stops) to treat the many bed wetters they had.

When I got back to the zoo, there were volunteers with zero medical training with stethoscopes around their necks, listening to chests, or maybe not, and then giving each patient ten amoxicillin capsules.

"We had to do something," they explained. "There were too many patients and you were off at the orphanage."

I didn't tell them they had the stethoscopes on backward. The earpieces should point forward. You can hear a lot more that way.

Doctors and nurses don't go on medical missions because they're good guys and gals trying to bring American know-how and medical advances to less fortunate people. Mostly we go because we like to do what we learned how to do in school. Most people who devote their lives to clinical medicine would do so for free if they could afford it.

When we got on the bus that was going to take us to the airport to get our flight home, local officials and police wouldn't let the bus move unless we gave them two hundred dollars American cash. We passed the hat.

The second time I went to Honduras went much better. Hondurans were in charge.

Never take more than twenty people on a mission. Don't call them missions. Put local people in charge and do what they say. Offering medical services for a week at a time should be illegal.

Death of an icon

> "Science is magic that works."
> KURT VONNEGUT JR.

Ten and a few years after Honduras, with a lot of pediatrics in between, my father died.

"If I should die, God forbid . . ." were the opening words in his yearly letter to me describing what he did and didn't want to happen when he died. It's amazing that a man who smoked two-plus packs of unfiltered cigarettes per day lived as long as he did and that, in the end, something else killed him. He claimed that doctors told him not to quit smoking, because it would be too great a shock to his system. He also claimed that his barrel-chested, chronic-coughing self didn't have any lung disease from smoking.

"Truly amazing, Dad." He wasn't a lot of fun to argue with.

One of my favorite episodes with my father was when we were on a stage together talking to Harvard students. A student started,

"Mr. Vonnegut . . . ?" My father turned to me as if I was supposed to answer. "Actually, I'm Doctor Vonnegut," I said.

For just a moment, the cultural icon looked stunned, and then he laughed.

Once, when he threw what would have been the winning dart in one of our family dart games, I called a foot fault. It had never been done before and he had the same stunned look.

A neurosurgeon resident at Bellevue Hospital referred to him as a cultural icon. I usually referred to him as Kurt if I referred to him at all. I loved him dearly but there was something about calling him "Dad" that didn't sound quite right. He was more like an unpredictable little brother, who might get himself, or me, or both of us, in trouble.

When my sisters and I started calling him "Junior" he went to the trouble of legally changing his name to just "Kurt Vonnegut."

Along with his instructions about no church, no religion, no public event celebrating him, his life, or his work, he was very clear that there should be no extraordinary measures taken to prolong his life—no CPR, intubation, ventilator, dialysis, resuscitation, etc.

What most living wills say is "If I'm dying, let me die," but even with very clear, simple written instructions—signed, witnessed, and notarized—what actually happens is often quite different. Ultimately, he was resuscitated, intubated, ventilated, artificially fed and hydrated, and treated for infections he probably didn't have. If his kidneys had failed, he would have been dialyzed.

After falling and hitting his head, my father passed through the surgical ICU suite reserved for President George Bush, who wasn't using it at the time and thankfully never did. Along with the high-tech medical equipment that was keeping my father alive, the twenty-fifth floor of the magnificent steel-and-glass tower had a very nice unobstructed view of the East River that my father never woke up to see.

I felt bad for the neurosurgery team. There was nothing surgical for them to do and they struggled to find not-awkward things to say. I would have given anything to have him wake up and make wry observations they wouldn't know how to take, maybe about the nice view or the fact that he was in the ICU bed reserved for President Bush if anything happened to him in NYC.

"Quite an honor."

It took several weeks for him to die, mostly because of medical interventions no one felt that they had any real choice over. There are downsides to being an icon.

Another doctor asked me, "What was it like to grow up with an icon for a dad?" Uncertainty about when to stop trying to save someone's life can happen to anyone but there was something about the patient being famous that upped the ambivalence ante. Who would want to be known as the doctor who "lost" an icon? I'm sure that without my father's special rank, he wouldn't have ended up in the special surgical ICU bed with its floor-to-ceiling glass windows looking out over the East River.

"This is actually the surgical ICU bed reserved for President Bush if anything happens to him when he's in New York."

"Yeah. That's what your senior resident said."

"Where'd you go to medical school?"

"Harvard."

"Nice."

Eighty-four-year-olds with brain injuries don't do well. After you get to be a certain age, just about everything that happens to you is permanent.

Knowing how and when to let a patient go isn't easy, especially once you've saved their life a few times and they're stable but ventilator dependent. Even with the full and certain knowledge that there's no meaningful hope, who wants to be a firing squad of one? Ultimately, we had to transfer my father to a different hospital that would allow us to carry out his wishes as best we knew them. We took him off the ventilator and as my father's son, I couldn't help saying, "I hope he hasn't changed his mind about the no-extraordinary-measures thing."

Among my father's heroes was Ignaz Semmelweis, M.D. Typical for my father's heroes, Ignaz's story doesn't end well. Semmelweis figures out and proves that childbirth fever, which was killing thousands of women shortly after they delivered their babies, was caused by doctors not washing their hands before examining their patients. Eventually this worked out well for the rest of the world in the form of cleaner, safer medical care. It also made childbirth a far less dangerous event.

For suggesting that doctors might be causing disease, Ignaz was pilloried and hounded out of his profession. He lost his license and hospital privileges, was shunned by his colleagues, driven mad, and beaten to death in a psychiatric hospital at the age of forty-seven. You can't make stuff like this up.

My father had an odd relationship with my mental illness. He seemed fascinated and a little jealous. Even though he knew it was a very painful biochemical screw up that didn't have much poetry or meaning, he came close to romanticizing it. When he was hospitalized briefly for swallowing pills, I told him he was doing a lousy imitation of someone with mental illness. Because he was Kurt Vonnegut, he got away with it. He didn't know shit about the voices.

"There's a really good neuro-rehab in New Jersey that takes ventilator-dependent patients."

"Wake up, Dad. I can't believe you're missing this. President Bush's ICU bed . . . Nice view of the East River . . . Neuro-rehab in New Jersey that accepts ventilators . . . Cultural icon . . ."

"Neuro-Rehab in New Jersey" could have been the title of one of his short stories.

". . . there's still quite a bit of cortical activity."

"Great. Dad, you have cortical activity."

So we made a playlist of all his favorite songs, mostly jazz from the forties and fifties, plus the Beatles, which we played at medium-high volume whenever nothing else was going on. When we were finally able to take him off the ventilator, he had been on it for four weeks. It's not impossible that he was looking at an eternity of hellfire and saying, "No, no, no, please don't take me off the vent," but I doubt it.

In high school and college, there are people who wonder what's the big deal about reading and maybe about life in general. They read a Kurt Vonnegut book or story and something clicks; they become part of something bigger than themselves and it feels good. He made people feel less lonely.

He was and is a gateway drug to the world of reading. I wish he had still been alive when I cut off part of my thumb with a table saw. He would have been jealous. My mother would have just winced in pain.

I'm now astounded and amazed by the beauty and quantity of my father's work. I didn't see it that way until after he'd been dead a few years. Maybe I was busy being nervous about what inappropriate or provocative thing he might do next that I might have to explain or forgive. My sister Edie and I visited him in the burn unit several years before he died, after he set the top floor of his townhouse on fire by falling asleep with a lit cigarette in his hand. There was mostly a lot of smoke and no real fire or flames. He had no burns on his face or body but was admitted for smoke inhalation.

It's not as if his lungs hadn't had practice with this smoke. Whether it's cigarettes or a fire in the building, smoke is smoke. A few days off in a burn unit must feel like life on a more hospitable planet. A planet where you have to smoke two and a half packs of cigarettes is different from one where you don't.

His O$_2$ saturation numbers on the monitor were running about what Edie's and mine probably were. He was heavily sedated, on a ventilator, breathing 28 percent oxygen, and Edie and I thought it was funny, in a touching way, how close we could get to him and even touch his face without him moving.

"Will he remember this?" Edie asked.

"Not a chance in hell."

If not George Bush or Kurt Vonnegut Jr., I am pretty sure Bellevue would have used that ICU bed for someone else. If you want medical care to be there for you when you need it, it's good to let doctors practice on other people and not get too rusty.

Medicare paid for most of my father's care. Bellevue Hospital is one of the best hospitals in the world. Like other great hospitals, they got that way by devoting themselves to science and taking care of whatever patients came their way. Sorting sick people has always been more trouble than it's worth.

My mother died twenty years earlier in hospice after a five-year battle with stage 4 ovarian cancer. Throughout her life, she lived very modestly and had managed to save and invest some money, which she had hoped to be able to leave to her children. Medical care got all but $20,000 of it, and that $20K was gobbled up by lawyers overseeing her estate. For me it wasn't about the money as much as it was about my mother, one year short of being eligible for Medicare, spending most of what little time and energy she had left with co-payments, balance billing, receipts and bills from hospitals, surgeons, oncologists, and doctors she couldn't remember meeting. I regularly apologized to her and my siblings about my profession. She didn't achieve the blessing of unconsciousness until the last week of her illness.

"It feels like I'm being held upside down and shaken, to make sure they get every last penny," said my mother.

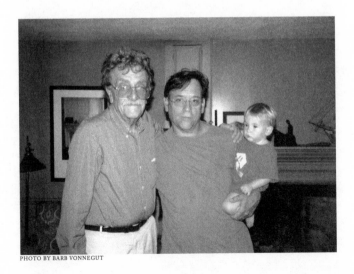

PHOTO BY BARB VONNEGUT

A man steps on a nail

> "Consumption is a double tragedy: what begins in inadequacy will end in deprivation."
> MARSHALL SAHLINS, **economist**

Urgent care centers, minute clinics, and other retail medical care outlets can provide good care but they often over test, over diagnose, overtreat, and overcharge. Also worth noting is that urgent care centers and minute clinics put local hospitals and community doctors out of business. A higher and higher percentage of medical care is delivered by doctors, NPs, or PAs who have never seen the patient before and will never see the patient again. Even at good hospital-based primary care practices, more and more of the care is of the "one and done" variety.

Especially on the weekends and holidays, more of our patients are going to urgent care centers or minute clinics. We're on call 24-7 and have regular hours Saturdays and sometimes see patients on Sundays and holidays. Most of our patients know this but don't want to be told to come in Monday for minor complaints because that might make them miss work. With digitalized medical care and billing, doctors are interchangeable parts—a doctor is a doctor, a patient is a patient, a throat culture is a throat culture.

"Can I see your insurance card, please?"

Urgent care centers pick and choose whom they treat. Inconvenient patients (i.e., those who are "too sick" or uninsured) can be sent home or to an emergency room. Ninety-plus percent of patients have no defense against bad or indifferent medical care. Most people figure that doctors know what they're doing until they themselves need care for a nontrivial illness, at which point many of them become a little more knowledgeable and fussy.

I shouldn't be taking care of friends and family, and mostly I don't, except when my friends and family are getting abysmally bad care that really might kill them. I have bitten my poor tongue almost in half many times. It seems to me that the need for tongue biting and the need for me to say something about the medical care of friends and family are much greater than they used to be, mostly because friends and family have such a hard time getting good primary care or reasonable advice about what they should do when they're sick.

I've recently had two lifelong friends die of liver failure, hepatitis C, alcohol, and poor insurance coverage almost exactly a year apart. I couldn't help thinking that maybe this or that could have been tried. It's probable that none of the possible treatments I thought about would have helped, but it seemed as if no one cared enough to at least think about trying something.

A cousin I grew up with almost got a colostomy he didn't need. "Get your ass out of that hospital and to MGH. They know you're coming," I sputtered.

A fireman fell off a ladder, cracked two ribs, collapsed a lung, and was having trouble breathing. He called me from a local ER after waiting for two hours and I said, "Yes. This could be serious. Are you getting more and more out of breath?" His wife then called an ambulance, which took him to another ER, where they gave him some oxygen, did a chest x-ray, and put in a chest tube.

Stepping on a nail shouldn't be a big deal. I have a friend named Rick who's a Vietnam vet who taught people how to jump out of planes and not die. He's a former division 1 college basketball player who stays in shape by going to the gym regularly and running every day. He raised three sons as a single father and was still working full time at the age of seventy-five.

I hadn't heard from Rick in a while when he called me out of the blue.

"I stepped on a nail and it hurts like hell. We just had the roof redone. It was one of those big galvanized flat-headed nails. Must have been sticking straight up. I feel like an idiot. I think I should go to the urgent care center. What's the worst that could happen?"

In my experience, it's bad luck to ask, "What's the worst that could happen?"

"Did you call your primary care guy?"

"Yeah, but the on-call doctor never called me back."

I really didn't think urgent care could screw up a minor puncture wound. I thought they'd just give him a tetanus shot and call it a day.

The doctor at urgent care decides to incise the wound and screws up the local anesthetic so the incision hurts much more than the original puncture wound. The doctor reassures Rick that the pain will lessen and that the incision will prevent infection and pain in the long run. Rick is put on oral antibiotics and an antibiotic ointment. "Call us if it doesn't feel better in the morning," the doctor says.

Come morning, the foot feels quite a bit worse. There's swelling and a bit of drainage on the gauze dressing so Rick, a good and compliant patient throughout his ordeal, calls and goes back to urgent care, where they do a deeper incision that doesn't hurt as much this time, because they manage to do the local anesthetic right.

The next day the pain is worse and there's more drainage. With two visits and two surgical procedures behind them, urgent care calls it a day and sends Rick to the local emergency room. Rick is admitted to the hospital for IV antibiotics to "get on top of" any possible infection. The hospital goes all out with an x-ray, an MRI, and many, many blood tests. And they order an infectious-disease consult.

Rick calls me and brings me up to date. I'm horrified and wonder what I could have or should have done differently. I go visit Rick in the hospital. He looks ten years older and thoroughly wrung out. I'm hopeful the infectious-disease consult will bring some much-needed light to the situation. Hope springs eternal.

The ID consult thinks that maybe Rick doesn't have an infection, maybe it's gout, but before the rheumatology consultant can see him, Rick goes home on oral antibiotics just in case. Doing things "just in case" is another thing that often ends badly.

Three days later there's more pain and more swelling. Rick can't walk. He's readmitted to the hospital for more IV antibiotics. The rheumatologist is sure it's not gout. At this point Rick figures he must be dying and the doctors don't know what they're doing. Rick is sent home on IV antibiotics administered via an indwelling central-line catheter, which a nurse will come help him with twice a day.

✦　✦　✦

Two days later my phone rings. "Mark, my other foot is swollen. An infection can't jump from the left foot to the right, can it?"

"Here's the deal, Rick, you're going to call your son and have him take you to Mass General."

"By ambulance?"

"No, Rick, not by ambulance. You'll get there more quickly and safely if your son drives."

The hero of Rick's story was a third-year medical student who, unburdened by the need to enter things into an electronic medical record, took a thorough history and did a careful physical exam.

The medical student correctly determined that Rick had never had an infection, that he was dehydrated because of colitis, probably clostridium difficile, from all the antibiotics he took. He was also in kidney failure because of the antibiotics, which was why both his feet and ankles were now swollen. His liver enzymes were up for some unknown reason but would probably return to normal once all the other problems were straightened out.

There will always be mistakes and bad outcomes, but they didn't used to cost $50K. His kidneys, liver, and colitis got better, but the pain and swelling in his right foot and ankle didn't. He was diagnosed with complex regional pain syndrome by his primary care physician. The visit to urgent care, along with the $50,000 in medical costs, was paid for by Medicare. Above and beyond the money part of things, a vigorous, fully employed man was forced to retire on full disability.

Bouncing back is a young man's game.

There's nothing in Rick's billing, coding, or his electronic urgent-care or hospital records that indicates what an unnecessary and very expensive disaster his care was. The electronic part of his care and coding was perfect.

Stockholm Syndrome

Victims of abuse sometimes bond with their captors or abusers and come to believe that the abuser must be right. This pathological connection develops over the course of the days, weeks, months, or even years of abuse and usually when the victim loses hope.

Sixty years ago, what kept medical care honest and costs down was that patients paid directly for healthcare. If they weren't happy, they could and did vote with their feet and wallets. Doctors, along with having a professional commitment to put their patients first, knew that not seeing to the needs of their patients had economic consequences. With patients no longer in charge, healthcare has gone nuts. There is effectively no one in the picture who has any power or interest in controlling costs. The way home is to get up off our knees begging for crumbs and put the patients back in charge.

Eight-hour waits and impersonal, careless care in emergency rooms or elsewhere wouldn't have happened or been tolerated sixty years ago. I had my childhood cuts sewn up and broken bones set with a smile at Cape Cod Hospital.

We've gotten used to bad medical care. Patients, doctors, and hospitals believe that our utterly nuts, inefficient patchwork, third-party insurance system must be right. Theirs is the hand that feeds us. As things are now, without insurance we have no healthcare. It's far from clear how or when things will change.

Rick never complained once about the lousy care that damn near killed him. He was a little bewildered but grateful throughout. "The doctor's a really nice guy."

Frogs won't jump out of hot water if you bring it to a boil slowly enough. We have come to believe that gatekeeping, performance metrics, eight-hour waits in an ER, blizzards of pharmaceutical ads, most of our rural hospitals closed down, unaffordable insulin, and spending $4 trillion on not very good healthcare must be somehow OK. OK?

A single-payer system would solve many problems, but if we're not careful about how we set it up we could end up with care that's only a little bit or not at all better than what we have now. Being for or against commercial insurance or capitalism or socialism is worse than a waste of time. To keep our eyes on the prize and avoid pointless fights and arguments we need to stick to a simple standard: What is good for patients?

While at one time it might have been reasonable to assume

that financial incentives like co-payments or quality improvement initiatives would help doctors and patients make more cost-effective choices, the failure of any such system to control costs or improve quality even a little bit means it's time to try something else.

It's actually not that hard to figure out. Step one would be get rid of past innovations that have failed or actually made things worse. If we are serious about delivering value we have to either decrease the amount of money patients pay into the system or increase the amount of care they have access to. The last thing patients need is more gates. Getting rid of co-payments would be a good start.

Lost Arts

> "A dinosaur's lament
> Yes, those are real tears."
> ME

Doctors as old as I am are called dinosaurs. I hope it's meant affectionately.

I had teachers who were so good at taking histories and doing physical exams that it looked as if they were performing sacred magic; sacred magic that I wanted to learn how to do. I especially remember one teacher whose hands barely touched—almost hovered over—the patient's body. He was so careful and she was so still that she might have floated off the bed and maybe, probably, been cured of whatever disease she had. The medical students were quiet. Maybe the whole hospital was quiet. The world paused. A careful physical exam makes a patient feel cared for, and feeling cared for is no small thing.

Autopsies are done much less often than they used to be. But when they are done it turns out that 20-plus percent of the time the patient didn't die from what the doctors thought he or she had. Without an accurate diagnosis, doctors are truly flying blind, and evidently they're flying blind a lot.

You can't do a good physical exam and punch data into a computer at the same time; you can't take a good history that way either. Listening to what the patient says is how doctors make correct diagnoses most of the time. The physical exam, x-rays, and blood tests can be useful but usually just confirm what you already know from what the patient told you. Patients, especially if you haven't seen them before, feel shortchanged if you don't do at least a little bit of a physical exam. If you can be quiet long enough, the patient will tell you what's wrong. It's very much in their best interest for you to get things right.

Over half the patients I see in follow-ups for ear infections diagnosed in the ER or urgent care have perfect eardrums that couldn't have been infected at any point in the recent past, let alone yesterday. They flat out never had an ear infection. Ninety-nine percent of the time they were treated with antibiotics they wouldn't have needed even if they did have an ear infection. Not all ear infections need to be treated with antibiotics. Explaining choices is another thing most emergency room doctors, even good ones, don't have time to do.

So many babies and kids are diagnosed with ear infections because time is short and no one else can see what the ER doc is seeing or not seeing with an otoscope. Maybe the eardrum looks a little red; maybe it doesn't. The babies are almost always crying, especially after a two-to-four-hour wait. Crying turns eardrums reddish and gives the doctor a "what's the harm" way to end the visit with a prescription.

Making convenient diagnoses and using unnecessary medications is a "whatever gets you through the night" kind of thing. There are always sicker patients who need to be seen. There's no time or incentive to diagnose minor diseases like ear infections correctly. Nothing bad happens if you get it wrong—except perhaps to your sense of self, if your self is paying attention.

For every eight-hour shift a doctor works, the powers that be dictate that the doctor must spend two to three hours more banging out their electronic-medical-record notes, which will never even be read. Thankfully, most patient-doctor encounters are not matters of life and death.

Second-guessing dinosaurs who went to medical school is a very expensive waste of time.

Not Fair

"If life was fair, Elvis would be alive and
all the impersonators would be dead."
JOHNNY CARSON

"I'm glad we're catching her up on her immunizations," I said.
I'd known the family for a long time, which always makes things
easier, more interesting, and more fun.

"I don't want to use the combinations. Can we divide them up?"
the mother asked.

"It costs a lot more, has the same side effects, makes no sense,
means giving her four needles instead of one. I hate needles," I
replied.

"I still want to break them up. I'll pay the extra," said the mother.

"You have to order them special from the pharmacy. It's about
a thousand dollars. She and you are both here now. Let's just get
it done," I offered.

Silence.

I turn to the seven-year-old. "Your mother wants you to get

four shots. I want you to get one. I went to medical school, your mother didn't. How many shots do you want?"

"One," said the angelic, forever-beloved child.

"That's not fair," said her mother.

Two against one. She got one shot.

She still smiles, shakes her head, and says, "Not fair," with her eyes when she sees me. And I say, "I'd do it again in a heartbeat," with my eyes back to her.

All's fair in love, war, and pediatrics.

Pee

Spending time with patients means you don't have to make things up if you don't want to. The truth is enough.

"You have to pee in a cup."

   "What's wrong with your bathroom?"

Wisdom from the Mouths of Babes

"Are you sure he needs an x-ray?" asked the mother of a ten-year-old boy.

"Mom, if Doctor Vonnegut says I need an x-ray, I need an x-ray."

Bless you, child.

Earwax and Warts

It used to just be part of the visit. If I couldn't see the eardrum because there was wax in the way, or if wax was blocking the ear canal, making it hard for the patient to hear, I removed the wax with a tiny metal or plastic loop doohickey.

Thanks to insurance, removing earwax is now a separately coded, billed, and reimbursed procedure. "Well, sure, I could dig the wax out of there, but it's going to cost extra" wouldn't fly in a cash-based system.

There's a lot of earwax out there and a lot of money—one hundred dollars and up per ear—to be made digging it out. There's also a lot of money to be made freezing warts and other skin lesions instead of letting them die a natural death, as well as other "sort of surgical" procedures.

Doctors are besieged with advertisements for lab equipment, tests, and machines that are "revenue enhancers." You can bill extra for them to make up the few thousand dollars they cost, then the extra money is all yours.

Digging out earwax for the money probably isn't why you went to medical school. Or buying fancy machines you don't really need just because they are revenue enhancers.

But without gaming the system it's hard to stay in business. Maybe the community hospitals that went under in the last thirty years should have done more earwax.

When insurers took control of pediatrics, they told us, "Look how much you're going to get paid for earwax and warts, along with the twice as much you get paid for well baby visits."

Therapy

The smartest thing I ever did in my practice was hire social workers and have them on site. There's never any lack of things for them to do, including listening to teenagers explain why they hate therapy. There is a peculiar aloneness to each and every one of us.

"I tried it once and I absolutely hate therapy."

"Great. I don't like it much myself, but I just happen to have a therapist here so you can explain to her why you hate therapy. If you can get better without talking to someone, I'm all for it. One hundred percent. And please come back and tell me how you managed to get un-depressed, un-anxious, un-flunking French, or whatever else without talking to anyone so I can tell others. Try running two miles each day, eating better, doing your homework, and not smoking marijuana. We might be able to get you out of having anything to do with a therapist altogether."

Negotiation

"Billy, your mother thinks that maybe you're depressed. Your grades are way down, you're not doing homework. She found marijuana in your room."

"Marijuana is legal now."

"Doesn't mean it's good for you. I'm not up on the law, but I don't think it's legal for fourteen-year-olds. She says you're not going out with your friends or doing sports anymore. Do you think you might be depressed?"

Blank face of bland indifference.

"Lots of fourteen-year-olds get depressed, and there are lots of ways to get un-depressed. Would you be willing to change your diet? Lift weights? Join a boxing gym? Talk to someone? Stop smoking marijuana for a week? Do something other than video games and YouTube?"

Nothing, nothing, nothing.

"Is there anything your parents could do that might make things better?"

"They could stop bugging me."

"That's a start. Anything else? Do you have enough money? Do you care about money? I might be able to get your parents to pay you to do some of the positive things I mentioned. It's not like joining the military or getting married. If doing positive stuff doesn't help you feel better, you can just quit."

"I have enough money."

"That's too bad."

"What?"

"Nothing. It's just that your having plenty of money takes away my favorite option. I sometimes throw in my own money. Do you have any pets?"

"No. Why?"

"I'm about out of ideas and I was wondering whether getting you a puppy might cheer you up?"

Smile. "But my parents would never go along with that."

"Would you take care of the puppy, walk the puppy?"

"Yes, but my parents would never—"

"I'll bet if you were willing to clean up your diet, do your homework, give the weed a break, and get a little more exercise, they would consider a puppy. Plus, I'll throw in that they have to stop bugging you."

"No way."

"Yes way. Let me go get them."

I return with the parents and start with the puppy idea.

"We couldn't possibly . . ."

"I told you." Billy drifts back to indifference.

"Let me finish. If Billy is willing and able to eat better, run two miles a day, do his homework, and stop smoking marijuana, wouldn't that make you at least more willing to be willing to be willing to be at least open to thinking about getting a puppy? And he'll clean up his room. And as long as he's holding up his end of the deal, you guys will have to stop bugging him and telling him what to do. OK?"

The parents often look a little hurt and puzzled.

"Let's meet again in a month to see how things are going. And if it's OK with you, Billy, we'll do a drug test to see how that's going for you. It's easier to start marijuana than to stop."

There are many situations in which drug tests aren't really necessary: if your mother brings you in for testing; or if you bring in someone else's urine for the test; or if your urine is closer to room temperature than body temperature; or if you start talking about the Constitution and illegal search and seizure; or if, after leaving some pee in a cup in the bathroom, you leave the office in a huff to wait for your mother in the parking lot rather than chat with me; or if your face falls at the mention of drug tests. Patients are nearly always grateful when I defer testing and suggest that we try for clean urine in a few weeks. Being relieved when I say that is also a good sign that we don't need to do the test.

During follow-up I focus on whether the parents are upholding their end of the bargain and being less annoying and controlling and whether the patient has given any thought to what kind of a puppy to get if allowed. I call it a therapeutic alliance.

Jamal

> "One of the most important gifts a parent can give a child is the gift of accepting that child's uniqueness."
>
> FRED ROGERS

Jamal is currently a very big, strong, six-foot-four, 240-pound autistic but verbal young man who outweighed his mother by the time he was ten. She was raising Jamal as a single mom.

Not now but back then, Jamal could become violent. One day his mother was driving and he got free of his seatbelt and started punching her. She pulled off the road to defend herself and not get into an accident. The police came and brought Jamal and his mother to an emergency room where he was sedated with medication and an admission to a child psych unit was arranged.

So far so good, and there was even appropriate care, but day after day the psych unit was unable to free up a bed. Jamal and his mother spent five days in the ER where they couldn't do much for him but keep him on sedatives and take his blood pressure and temperature. Jamal calmed down and was finally admitted to the psych hospital where, they confirmed his autism diagnosis but couldn't make up their minds about medication. Two days after admission, they sent him and his mother home with a prescription for a medication with serious side effects, like obesity and diabetes, just in case it might help. "And follow-up with your pediatrician." A hospital for children that puts children on serious medications that might help and doesn't see them back for follow-up isn't quite right.

Among the other things ERs are not good with is mental illness. Mentally ill people, along with other unfortunates with nowhere to go, clog up ERs, making it hard for them to be ready for accidents, life-threatening illnesses, and injuries. Hospitals used to have psychiatric beds, but these have been mostly eliminated because they aren't cost effective for the insurance companies. No one has ever thought that inpatient psychiatric hospitalization was a great option but sometimes there is truly no other option. Not having any beds doesn't make the patients or the problems go away.

Jamal had thick wavy hair halfway down his back. When he was twelve he decided to have his beautiful hair cut off and donated to a company that made wigs for chemotherapy patients. His hair probably made two or three wigs. There was something about donating his hair that changed Jamal into a sweet and very empathetic giant boy. He hasn't been violent since, which is a very good thing. He could take me out with one punch.

He hasn't needed medication, emergency rooms, or hospitals since he donated his hair.

The mother who wouldn't let me touch her baby

> "For, after all, how do we know that two and two make four? Or that the force of gravity works?"
>
> GEORGE ORWELL

Her logic was that, since she wouldn't let me immunize her baby, I needed to wear gloves to protect her baby from germs. She had listened carefully once or twice to my explanations about how immunization was the best way to go, then she looked at me politely and simply said, "No. Not today." I was a waiter whose suggestion had been rejected after being asked what I thought was best.

"The DTaP is very good today. We had someone with whooping cough in just this morning."

After the first few visits I just came into the room, carefully washed my hands, and put on gloves while she looked on approvingly. She couldn't have been more friendly and pleasant. Her baby actually got whooping cough when he was nine months old. Luckily it was a mild case and he did well. I wrongly assumed that she would then go along with immunizations.

I have no idea what she was like before having a baby. I believe she probably had always had eccentric opinions. I would be the last person to hold people's eccentric opinions against them. If we excluded parents with irrational ideas about their children, we'd be taking care of a few dozen patients at most.

We take care of people regardless of race, religion, socioeconomic status, or nutty ideas.

"My job is to tell you what science knows and what it doesn't know. I hope you'll come to trust us enough to let us immunize your baby."

"Thank you, Doctor. Not today."

My efforts to change her mind about immunization were fewer and farther between.

When the baby turned one, it was all of a sudden OK to immunize him, and I no longer had to wear gloves.

I look forward to staying tuned and seeing how their story, and others like it, play out over time.

Having schools, not pediatricians, give immunizations would cut costs and immunization refusal by half, at least. School nurses don't suffer fools and nonsense nearly as much as we do. I promise we pediatricians would find something else to do with the time; maybe teach medical students, read journals, and catch our breath.

Notes home from school

> "The consequences of an act affect the probability of its occurring again."
>
> B. F. SKINNER, the father of behavior modification

Chris's mother: "I've been getting notes home from his teacher. She says Chris doesn't pay attention, and she thinks he might have ADHD. Grades are fine. He has lots of friends, plays sports. Everything else is fine."

"So the problem here is mostly the notes coming home. Does he help out around the house? Is he mostly nice to you and the rest of the family?"

"Mostly."

"Last year and the year before there were no notes?"

"Right. No notes."

I look over at Chris, wearing the beatific smile of a twelve-year-old boy who has completely and utterly befuddled the woman who gave birth to him.

"Chris, you're a smart kid. Do you think it's possible for you to act in such a way that your teacher stops sending home those notes? I bet that your mother would be willing to pay money to not have to deal with them."

"Really?"

"The details would be up to you and your mom and you wouldn't get money for just a few weeks of no notes. To get serious money, it would have to be no notes for like the rest of the year."

"Mom, what do you think?"

"I'm thinking."

"All you have to do is sit up front, look at the teacher most of the time and pretend to care. You don't have to really care."

"How much money?"

"Ask your mother. And clean up your diet and get a little more exercise? It's worth a try."

The notes stopped coming home for a couple of years. ADHD is a real thing and teachers are often right. Two years after the above meeting, when Chris started high school, he was diagnosed with ADHD. I'm glad he's doing well on medication, but I'm not even a little sorry that I "missed" his ADHD when he was twelve.

Having trouble sitting still, having more energy than most people, seeing things a little differently, being bored when things are boring, having impulses not all of which are good, looking out the window and wondering what's going on out there can all be adapted to if you're an adult, but not so much if you're trying to survive grades 1 through 12.

Malcolm

> "The opposite of love is not hate,
> but indifference."
>
> WILHELM STEKEL, M.D.

A perfectly healthy eight-year-old boy woke up suddenly unable to move or feel anything from the waist down. His mother rushed him in to see us. We thought it was a very rare inflammation of the spinal cord called transverse myelitis and sent him by ambulance into the pediatric service of a major teaching hospital. The paralysis from transverse myelitis sometimes gets better but usually not, especially if there's no improvement early on. The hospital agreed with our diagnosis, but once he was stable, the family took him down to Johns Hopkins for a second opinion. They diagnosed him as having an even rarer stroke of the spinal cord. Somehow a clot had broken free and come to block the artery that fed a small segment of his spinal cord. This severed all communication between his brain and his lower body and paralyzed him from the waist down. The paralysis and loss of feeling is unfortunately permanent.

155

Today Malcolm is in a wheelchair and is truly one of the nicest people I know. He is a classical guitarist who will probably end up playing professionally. We see Malcolm not infrequently for complications of his paralysis, like urinary-tract infections and bedsores, but the most time-consuming thing we do for Malcolm and his family is fill out reams and reams of paperwork certifying that his wheelchair and other things his paralysis makes necessary are, in fact, "medically necessary." My medical home-care coordinator, Joan, and I wonder if the insurance people are hoping we give up or screw up in a way that will allow them to wash their hands of Malcolm.

Dear Insurer,

Malcom still needs a wheelchair and Maggie still has no left leg.

Coach Smith

"So we go to medical school
To make what is known available
To those who need it
And all they hear is why and how
The doctor won't see you now."

ME

Nephrotic syndrome occurs when the kidneys, which are constantly filtering your blood to remove toxins and wastes, fail to capture and recirculate albumin, the protein that acts like a sponge to keep water and salt in your circulation. Your blood is only about 40 percent red and white blood cells. The rest is water, salt, and protein. Without enough protein in your veins and arteries, the water and salt leak out of your capillaries into the rest of your body and you blow up like a balloon. Sorry for the long explanation.

Nephrotic syndrome for Coach Smith started with his feet and ankles getting a little puffy. If he pressed his ankle with a thumb it made a dent that stayed a dent for a countable number of seconds. And then he got a lot puffy.

Coach Smith had been a professional tennis player and a semiprofessional baseball player, a million years ago. He had a slightly scrambled way of putting words together, and he was a lot of fun to talk with, even if I had trouble following what he said. We had lived together back in the seventies when I was trying to write a book and get into medical school and he was writing music and playing in local bars. Back then, he had a Prince Valiant haircut, bangs and all. I went out with him to the bars once, figuring he knew how to talk to women. I remember asking him, "What about that one?" or "What about them?" a couple of times until it dawned on me that my handsome, poised friend was no better at meeting women than I was. He talked a good game.

Fast-forward forty years, and my friend Coach Smith—which is actually how he refers to himself on his answering machine—has coached three state championship tennis teams and is living half the time here on Cape Cod and half in Hawaii, with his new wife. He's still writing music and gives me saxophone parts to play, but I have to tone it down and not go all wild on him. Anyway, he calls to say his foot is sore and swollen and blistered and "probably infected." He'll be home soon and I can check it out. "Meanwhile, can you call in some antibiotics?"

Probably shouldn't have, but I called in some antibiotics. He's beaten me down before and gotten me to treat him for bronchitis against my better judgment. Treating friends and family at all is against my better judgment.

The foot got better but was still swollen. The pictures he sent me were out of focus, but it didn't look like an infection, maybe a bad sunburn. He'd be home soon. Anything that gets better in less than two weeks, whether or not the antibiotics had anything to do with it, is my kind of disease.

He comes home to Cape Cod on schedule and, within a week, is in the local ICU, out of breath, with chest pain and generalized edema, including two very swollen feet. It turns out he has the aforementioned nephrotic syndrome. Instead of behaving like a sensible person and holding on to his albumin, he's pissing it all away. When I visit him in the ICU, he's gained about forty pounds and looks old and very tired. His wife says he's lucky that she met him when he was still handsome.

Nephrotic syndrome often responds to steroids. Happily, the steroids work and Coach Smith briefly returns to 90 percent of his old self. And then the steroids don't work, and then they work but a little less than the first time, and then they don't work and don't work again and again. He's now moon faced, humpbacked, and afflicted with all the other side effects of the prednisone that was initially his friend. Every time his local nephrologist tries to ween him from steroids, the swelling and the rest of his symptoms come back. And the nephrologist, who gives Coach less than five minutes of attention after he's waited twenty minutes or more, prescribes more prednisone. My fit, athletic friend has turned into a 240-pound water balloon.

Coach is a Vietnam vet. I urge him to go to the VA for a second opinion. He says they'll make him wait too long and that he doesn't trust them anyway. He's now in a wheelchair; a water balloon in a wheelchair.

Part of my problem is that I know at least a little bit about almost everything and have faith that, with a little time and a little literature, I can figure out the rest, which is how I, as a pediatrician, have ended up with some sixty-, seventy-, eighty-, and even ninety-year-old patients. It's really the fault of other doctors, who seem to be taking lousier and lousier care of my friends.

Doctors used to do a better job of doing their jobs. They used to be more curious. They used to want to get it right. As a profession, we've been whipped—"Yeah, yeah, yeah, but you still shouldn't be taking care of adult patients, especially ones you know," replied my wife.

"If their own goddamned doctors would just do their jobs, I wouldn't have to," I fumed back to my wife.

Problem number two is that lots of people I grew up with don't have health insurance. Insurance status didn't used to determine what kind of care you got. Suboptimal insurance is a relatively new disease that makes all other diseases worse. It's a disease that most of the rest of the world has figured out how to cure.

Nephrotic syndrome is actually something I know quite a bit about, because it happens not infrequently with kids, especially the "minimal change nephrotic syndrome" subtype, which is what Coach Smith had. I thanked him for at least coming up with a pediatric disease this time.

What I know about nephrotic syndrome is that when it relapses over and over again and the steroids become less and less effective, a small dose of a chemotherapy drug—there are at least two that can be effective—often puts the patient into long-term remission. I thought the nephrologist should have known this and given it a try, like, yesterday. But for over a year she remained loyal to prednisone and damn near killed Coach Smith.

Things continued to go downhill. His wife, Terry, called me and said that he was finally willing to get another opinion. We got him an appointment at MGH to see one of the nephrologists.

"Do you know him?"

"No, but that's OK, because they actually know what's going on at MGH and, amazingly, ask for help if they don't."

It was touch and go getting him into my father-in-law's old Lexus.

"How are we going to do this?" Terry asked when we got him into the wheelchair and out the back door.

"Maybe a forklift and a really big tub of Vaseline."

We got him to MGH, parked in front, slid him out of the car and into his chair with some help from security people, and got him into the building and up the elevator. We waited a few minutes before being seen by the nephrologist who knew what was going on and prescribed the drug we had used frequently during my residency at MGH. Over the next three months, Coach recovered from his nephrotic syndrome and his indifferent, incurious, unscientific medical care. He'll have to take a small amount of medication for the rest of his life but is back to teaching tennis, running five miles a day, spending winters in Hawaii, and writing music. It shouldn't be so hard to get access to the science and care our ancestors meant for us to have.

The kind of medical care Coach Smith received is zombie care. Zombies are hard to kill and they eat brains. Fewer and fewer patients seek care, which is less and less worth seeking, and this will mean more and more zombies. Zombie care works out well for the insurance industry and often pays better than "real" care.

Watching friends and family get bad care is like watching a train wreck in slow motion. At least Coach Smith did me the favor of getting well and going back to being his nutty, thick-headed, music-writing, recently married, blessedly normal-functioning-kidney self. And he has an MGH nephrologist to talk to.

Now, Coach Smith and I talk a lot about the Red Sox. He's optimistic that Chris Sale will be an ace pitcher again soon. I'm not so sure. Sale could definitely use a little more body fat, and skinny pitchers make me nervous.

Cutting

Sometimes it's about DNA, but mostly, we are what we do.

Patients didn't used to cut themselves. The careful, deliberate, superficial, just-deep-enough-to-draw-blood cutting of oneself was something that seemed to have started among upper-middle-class suburban high school girls, then spread to middle school girls, then boys.

Cutting has very little to do with suicide. It has much more to do with identity and being part of a group. Cutters almost never kill themselves. Cutting has spread like a contagious disease on the internet, in schools, and among friends. It seems to have become almost a normal part of growing up.

Cutting is the opposite of passion and lashing out. There's a ritual to it. The cuts are evenly spaced, just deep enough to draw blood. It's like trying both to not hurt yourself and to hurt yourself at the same time. It takes presence of mind, concentration, a steady hand, and good coordination.

Parents and other adults aren't nearly as shocked by cutting as they used to be. They still go crazy but not as much. Cutting is more and more a way to get attention and ask for help. Most cutters have a bland attitude and flat affect, and they seem as if they could care less about what I or their parents think. I hope the apparent indifference is posture, and I mirror back that I care even less than the less that they care, which seems to intrigue them. Anything to start a conversation.

It's not unlike the discipline required by anorexia. As there is in cases of depression and anxiety, there's a brain chemistry part of it and a peer-group identification part of it.

When cutters tell me cutting makes them feel alive or less anxious or gets them out of depression, I tell them we have more effective ways to deal with anxiety and depression symptoms. "Why don't you try it our way for a few weeks and see whether you feel better?"

Phone calls are how most referrals to psychiatrists and other specialists used to work. I'd tell the specialist what I was worried about, they'd see the patient within a week or so and call me back to tell me what they thought. It was very direct, efficient, and much safer than what goes on today.

The real news to many cutters is that there are adults who aren't afraid of them or their cutting and who care enough about them to want to see them come back again. Therapy works really well for these kids if they're willing to give it a try. Thank God for our social workers, who have great patience and understanding.

Self-harm and suicide are among the problems I didn't expect to be dealing with as a primary care pediatrician. I thought I'd be doing ear infections, coughs, and fever with some asthma, pneumonia, vomiting, diarrhea, and rashes, and making sure more serious problems didn't sneak through. When cutting started to be a thing, I could call up a psychiatrist when a patient started cutting. The psychiatrist would see and take care of the patient that week or the next week. The current wait time to see a psychiatrist is six months. We should be ashamed.

I wish anorectics would just eat. They would feel better and good nutrition would help their anxiety. It's all about control combined with a distorted body image. Why don't you just take a walk or shoot some hoops or anything other than not eating or carefully cutting little lines on your arms? Just stopping the behavior would make life easier and better for them and me and their parents and all the other people who want them to stop cutting or start eating. Maybe not a cheeseburger, but try roasted cauliflower with yellow peppers, cherry tomatoes, and feta cheese.

Earlier in my career, I had a patient who had experienced a lot of trauma in her childhood. Cutting, which she said gave her relief, was among her problems. Like most of my patients back then who had serious emotional problems, I sent her to a psychiatrist whom I talked with from time to time. She made great progress, went back to college, was getting back into sports, and now had a decent boyfriend. She came to my office just to say "hi" and fill me in on how she'd been doing. After filling me in and thanking me for taking care of her, she turned to go, paused, turned back to me, and bared her forearms, which had some perfectly straight, fresh, superficial cuts.

"Is it all right if I still cut?"

"Are you still seeing Doctor Adams?" I asked hopefully.

Addiction

> "I can't stand the rain."
> TINA TURNER

No one grows up wanting to be an addict. I don't think of it as a choice as much as a lack of better choices, over and over again. My generation worked very hard to prove that drugs are bad for you. More recent generations should honor our sacrifices by not doing drugs. There's a grim lack of playfulness in how most people do drugs today.

The problem isn't that the current generation makes bad choices as much as it is that they don't have enough good choices. They don't have the naive optimism I grew up with, the assurance that working hard would pay off; onward and upward. And there's the not-insignificant fact that drugs make potential addicts feel better than they've ever felt before. "My prince has come."

There's nothing sadder and more tragic than losing a child to addiction. Unfortunately this is now a routine part of pediatrics no matter where you practice. These days I can diagnose addiction just by looking at a patient. The slightly goofy child you're used to seeing and taking care of is gone. Their baby-face cheeks are gone, they have a new pseudo-swagger. Sometimes I just cut to the chase and ask them how long they've been taking drugs. Sometimes they ask me how I knew.

Once upon a time I was offered cocaine. This was back when lots of people believed cocaine wasn't addictive. It made me chattier and more social. When I found out that I had consumed a hundred dollars' worth of cocaine, I was horrified. It wasn't worth one hundred dollars to be a little chattier and more social. I was also offered heroin by a rock-and-roll band I had played with a few times and was thinking of joining. I turned down the heroin and didn't join the band.

When my cousin and his best friend smoked grass for the first time, they tasked me with writing down what happened and what was said so later they could compare their memories with my notes. Science at work.

My personal drug history is mild for the times I grew up in. Without knowing why, as a teenager I didn't trust drugs or myself. At that time, in those places and for me, drugs were a choice. I never even liked marijuana very much. My friends didn't push me to take drugs. I somehow knew that drugs would be worse for me than they were for other people long before I had a psychiatric diagnosis and had been hospitalized.

In the sixties, when people started taking LSD and other hallucinogens, it was because they didn't know what was going to happen. Today, when my patients and other young people start taking narcotics, they know what happens next and want it to happen: the warm hug. The thing they've been looking for has arrived.

It seems like a choice. It's easy to quit after the first and the second time you use a drug. You can put it down for a week or a month. Delusions of self-mastery and a lack of other things to do set you up for the next time, and the next, until you reach whatever your magic dose happens to be. If you don't have a passion for music or art or sports or theater or anything else, cashing in all your insecurities, worries, and anxieties for the life of an addict seems like a relative bargain.

Drugs are easy to start and easy to keep taking. If you take drugs and drink every day, how can you tell what they're doing to you?

A perfectionist is a hard thing to be. Caitlyn had been a gymnast and a dancer when she was younger. She was fifteen and needed a physical for sports. She complained about being "too fat" in spite of being athletic and thin. She felt that her friends didn't like her and that playing sports was all she had going for her. If you're an anxious kid in high school, sooner or later someone is going to give you oxycontin and maybe a beer to wash it down; the anxiety and the pain behind it goes away, along with the feeling that you're on a race to nowhere. More than a few kids gifted enough to earn athletic scholarships to college see sports as a job that saves their parents money. I would have killed to be that good an athlete for the sheer joy of it.

Some people can mess around with opioids for a relatively long time without getting into trouble with them and becoming dependent, but for Caitlyn the high felt so good that, in a month or so, she had a pill habit she couldn't afford. Heroin was the better, more manageable deal.

The perfectionist who used to get mostly As and had earned a full four-year athletic scholarship flunked out of UMass after two semesters. Opiates became her "drug of choice." She went home and waitressed until she lost that job. She was in detox after detox, rehab after rehab, and residential treatment after residential treatment. She doesn't call me anymore. Opiate users often stop crashing cars and getting arrested. It's almost as if they settle down and trade a bunch of little problems for one big one. Their race to nowhere is over.

I've seen families with the bad luck to have as many as three children with alcohol and drug problems. Near as I can tell, parents with multiple addicts aren't better or worse parents than any of the rest of us. The pain of losing a child or children to addiction is compounded by everyone else's assumptions that the parents must have done something wrong.

When marijuana takes over a child's life, it's somehow even more tragic because marijuana is supposed to be a less harmful, nonaddictive, and, now, legal drug. If it's not addictive, why are there so many teenagers and young adults who smoke it every day and can't stop? A child can seem so close to getting "it" right. A handsome, bright, gifted athlete stops caring about anything else and ends up twenty-nine years old, living in his parent's basement, pumping gas, and smoking weed every day. If he's not an addict, who is?

Robin was a runner. Halfway through high school she discovered that alcohol was a better mood stabilizer and much quicker cure for anxiety than Zoloft, which alcohol often is, until it isn't. When she was seventeen she was ending up in police stations and emergency rooms on a regular basis. Eventually it became a weekly thing. One of the bad things about being fourteen or seventeen and drinking heavily is that whatever happens when you're drunk seems normal or better than normal. Especially if your "normal" is feeling uncomfortable. The brash confident self that everyone seems to like better becomes the one you like better, too.

Robin started doing other drugs, which were also effective treatments for anxiety, and she started doing other things that were easier to do if you were drunk. She became a tough kid, which she really wasn't.

One Monday after she had ended up in the ER twice and in jail in protective custody once, her main complaint was that she was exhausted and hadn't slept for five days. She looked like hell.

There's an atypical antipsychotic medication that has a fairly dependable side effect of sleepiness, especially if someone hasn't taken it before. I wrote out a prescription. Thirty minutes later the mother called to tell me that the pharmacy wouldn't fill the prescription, because the insurance company would approve the medication only for someone with schizophrenia. After a long time on hold, I spent another not-inconsiderable while on the phone with one of the insurer's medical-utilization-review guys, who wouldn't budge. I wrote another prescription, but this time I wrote it for one of my nurses, who didn't have schizophrenia either but did have better insurance. They went to the pharmacy together, the prescription was filled, and Robin got some sleep.

She continued to drink and couldn't stay out of trouble. The girl who ran sub-five-minute miles and did well in school never went to college. She discovered the warm hug of IV opiates instead. She tried to get clean and sober several times but died of an overdose at home in the family living room while the rest of her family slept.

Whatever else we think about the opioid epidemic, it has been part of a successful business-as-usual plan for the pharmaceutical industry. Most addicts just want a chance to recover and sleep a little better.

Divide and Conquer

"Divide et impera."
JULIUS CAESAR

In the 1940s, '50s, '60s, and '70s, common purpose gave us a common language. The consensus built around science and what it meant to take good care of patients, along with boundless opportunities to work hard, made burnout impossible. We were all on the same side. What's happened since looks a lot like the tower of Babel. Patients, doctors, hospitals, and insurers have split and split and split into smaller and smaller groups beating each other's brains out. It's like the Harvard vs. Yale game with live ammunition.

It's hardly productive to have hospitals competing with hospitals for enhanced reimbursement, primary care competing with specialists, rich patients competing with poor patients, and so forth. We are moving toward being nations of one, which is exactly the opposite of where I thought science and service wanted us to go. To the extent our work is part of meaningless battles, why bother. The only group with any cohesion, capable of meaningful political activity, is the nurses.

Some big hospitals get 20 to 40 percent more money than smaller hospitals for the same operation or procedure. The former camaraderie and gentle teasing between doctors, different hospitals, and specialties are gone. Now they unsmilingly sit around polished granite tables in thousand-plus-dollar suits talking about "covered lives," which is insurance speak for people. Any new deal or change is scrutinized for whether it favors hospital-based or community-based providers. It's about money because it has to be.

Surgeons and specialists have always earned more than primary care doctors, but as the price of everything has gone up, those differences have gone from a manageable ~$50K to a can't-live-without-it ~$500K per year. It makes everyone grumpier and more nervous knowing that our incomes are dependent on the whims of insurers.

Enhanced reimbursement was forced on my practice. I get 20 percent more to treat an ear infection than a pediatrician with a less favorable PPO (preferred provider organization) contract. Everyone could use 10 to 20 percent more money but it's unusual to have someone put a gun to your head and make you take it.

Most of our grossly inflated overhead is about prior authorizations and other nonsense. We couldn't live without enhanced reimbursement.

As the costs of insurance and out-of-pocket expenses go up and up, patients who are most in need of medical care have to go without it. This is at the expense of their health, the public health, and our already overburdened safety-net programs. Many, many practices and hospitals have gone out of business.

When co-payments were first instituted, they added three dollars to each visit. It was supposed to be a cost-control measure that would make patients seek less unnecessary care. I felt sorry for the insurer involved, because they clearly didn't understand patients or medical care. When they came up with asthma quality improvement programs, I felt sorry for them because they knew so little about diagnosing or managing asthma. Americans who get sick or injured in Europe are astounded by how quickly they're seen and how little money it costs.

When we talk about repealing the Affordable Care Act, aka Obamacare, we're really talking about repealing medical care for patients who were formerly referred to as uninsured. We would be partially repealing penicillin, ambulance rides, and surgery. Presumably we would still provide some sort of care to people who collapse in front of a hospital.

"'Doc, this ten, fifteen, twenty dollars you're charging is like from stagecoach days. Do you see the cars the orthopedic guys are driving? You went to school with those guys. You and I know they're no smarter than you are. So let me explain how third-party billing can work for you."

"You're gonna get some computers, approximately thirty grand. No big deal. We can help with financing. And you get a biller type person, overhead goes up a little but overhead doesn't matter because of how much more money you'll be making. We will, of course, never, never in any way try to influence how you practice medicine. You're the guys who went to medical school."

"This employer-based medical insurance in pediatrics is going to be very big. Youse guys are like the last specialty to get in on it. Any pediatrician who doesn't go for it won't last long, because going to a doctor who takes insurance will be like it was free. Patients pay nothing to see you and we pay you a lot more than you're getting now."

Human greed is nothing new, but it wasn't supposed to happen to science and medical care. It wasn't supposed to happen to me.

When insurers took over pediatrics, it was gangster thuggery complete with leg breakers and deals we couldn't refuse.

For insurers, controlling how much money comes in and how much money goes out is like shooting fish in a barrel. When insurers enhanced reimbursement for patients with private insurance, it made taking care of underinsured patients less and less affordable. I'm paid much less to take care of Medicaid patients than I'm paid to take care of patients with "good" insurance. Every reimbursement enhancement comes with overhead enhancement.

What running a small primary care practice and having to balance the books has taught me is that there's really no difference between co-payments, deductibles, performance metrics, prior authorizations, asthma action plans, quality improvement initiatives, gold, silver, or bronze plans, closed or open panel, preferred provider organizations, and so forth. Without exception, all the above increase provider overhead and decrease access to care, especially if you're poor or live in a rural area or get sick a lot. All the quality metrics could be most easily met by finding a way to stop taking care of Medicaid patients or patients with asthma, cancer, or mental-health issues. What doctors and hospitals lose when they don't take care of complicated patients is their usefulness.

The Cost of
Not Caring

> "You cannot escape the responsibility
> of tomorrow by evading it today."
> ABRAHAM LINCOLN

Bad care is bad for everyone. There's no firewall between the cost of my medical care and your medical care. When we say that our insurance pays for something, we should bear in mind that it's more like a high-interest loan. Insurers collect trillions of dollars from us in the form of premiums and taxes. They pay out less than 80 percent to hospitals and other providers who are forced to compete against each other. The hospital construction and renovation boom of the past thirty years was a highly leveraged affair undertaken in the hopes of winning the enhanced-reimbursement game. It's all smoke and mirrors.

It's amazing to me that our medical care is as good as it is considering how little money we spend on patient care.

Not providing basic medical care to those who need it will inevitably cost us more than we save. The cost of everyone's medical care (currently 20 percent of the GNP) will continue to go up and up. Insurance will be less and less affordable. Everyone's access to care will continue to go down. Bankruptcies because of unaffordable medical care will continue to rise. Homelessness will continue to rise. Diabetics and asthmatics and patients with cancer or heart disease or mental illness don't just crawl into the bushes and die. The cost of the care they need goes up the longer it is put off.

Infections like hepatitis A, B, and C, tuberculosis, HIV, and COVID-19 will be harder and harder to control. The percentage of the population that is immunized will continue to fall. There will be less and less primary care, fewer and fewer hospitals, and more and more inappropriate emergency room utilization. Minute clinics and urgent care centers will become the new standard of care.

Unaffordable insulin doesn't just affect diabetics, we all end up paying for the extra amputations, ER visits, dialysis, and kidney transplants. Homelessness has a domino effect that leads to more tuberculosis, HIV, untreated mental illness, and hepatitis A, B, and C.

Without insurers to pay for them, there would be no $100,000 pills. Without $100,000 pills, there would be no exponential increases in the cost of care to justify ever-increasing premiums and the ever-increasing amounts of money they get to keep.

Our overhead crept up from 27 percent to 35 percent, and then to 50 percent. The same thing happened to other practices and hospitals as insurers began holding back money that we could get only if we met "performance" targets. The performance targets had nothing to do with performance. Quality improvement initiatives and other performance metrics are thinly veiled but effective punishments for taking care of sicker, more complicated, and poorer patients.

After two or three rounds of what amounted to a protection racket and loan sharking, we could no more survive without insurers than we could fly.

To mix in another metaphor: you can't win no-limit poker if the other guy has all the chips.

"Is this a game of chance?"
"Not the way we play it."

W. C. FIELDS

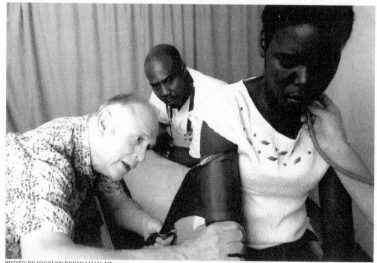

PHOTO BY JOCELYN BRESNAHAN, NP

Haiti

> "Since I do not believe that there should be different recommendations for people living in the Bronx and people living in Manhattan, I am uncomfortable making different recommendations for my patients in Boston and in Haiti."
>
> PAUL FARMER, M.D.

A few years after my father died, I went on a trip to Haiti to help out at a clinic run mostly by Haitians, which is definitely the way it has to be done if you want to do more good than harm. The clinic had been set up by a couple whose children were patients of mine in Boston. I once gave their mother a behavior-modification plan where she was supposed to give herself a gold star every time she didn't react to her daughter's temper tantrums. She tells me she went home fuming but the tantrums stopped. It's amazing the things people will forgive.

The family had been going back and forth to Haiti on a regular basis and I had always wanted to go. I went the week before Thanksgiving with another doctor, eight nurses, an educator, and a deaf priest.

Compared to Haiti, Honduras, where I had been on previous missions, is a country club. The twelve-mile car ride from the airport to the clinic took a little over four hours. There were small streams and rivers that were open sewers and people living in makeshift tents that had been there since the 2010 earthquake. The air was foul and palpably gritty. As we, ever so slowly, got further away from Port-au-Prince, the air and living conditions got a little better. The nurses, doctor, and priest I was traveling with had been there before. They had handkerchiefs tied over their noses and mouths. Their hair was wrapped up and covered. I was just taking it all in and was amazed at how gracious the Haitians were being about the worst traffic I'd ever seen. Back home, guns would have been pulled.

Up the mountain near the clinic, things were better still, with cinderblock houses, chickens, vegetable farming, and a few fruit trees. Whatever it was that made these people so poor, it wasn't their fault. They couldn't have been working harder. There were plenty of people who looked healthier than the average American. Those, of course, were the people well enough to be up and about, people who hadn't died in childhood and didn't have tuberculosis or AIDS.

In spite of healthy appearances, chronic diseases run rampant in Haiti and are a big part of what keeps Haitians and Haiti poor; poverty was at the root of their infectious diseases.

It's very, very hard for a Haitian to finish high school, let alone go to college. If they go to medical school, it's usually in Cuba. Medical care seems to be what Cubans do best. There were always teenagers and young adults hanging out and helping out at the clinic. They spoke excellent English and French and Creole. They often served as our translators. Several of them were musicians who had made a video of their band playing at a local church dance. They were good. They were smart, charming, energetic kids who would succeed in a heartbeat if you could smuggle them out of Haiti and into New York, Montreal, or maybe New Orleans. The poorer a place is, the harder it is to achieve escape velocity.

We had virtually no lab facilities, no x-rays, and not enough medications, but we did the best we could with what we had. The Haitians were very proud of their clinic. Suboptimal equipment and medications and poverty be damned.

Every evening, after dinner, the twelve volunteers went around the table describing what their day had been like and its most memorable moment. The priest, who was very deaf, led us in a prayer before the meal and the daily reflection. I initially thought of this as a candy-canes-unicorns-and-rainbows, unnecessary, team-building, rah-rah thing to do, but quickly got into it and enjoyed getting to know, learning about, and feeling part of the team; pretty good for a non-joiner.

There was a large deck overlooking the valley below, where we sat in giant rocking chairs, watched the sun go down, and listened to voodoo drums. Our Haitian staff said that, like a lot of Haiti, the mountain was Catholic during the day and voodoo by night, and there wasn't any real conflict. I joked about sneaking into a voodoo ceremony, and the Haitians smiled a little once they were sure I was kidding. I wish I was that brave.

The priest and I got along well. We were the only males on the trip so we bunked down in what was usually a dormitory with a trickling shower, which we kindly shared with the women. A deaf snoring priest would have been the perfect person to confess my sins to. I sometimes wished I'd been raised Catholic, because so many of my friends were Catholic and it would have given me something to accept or reject.

"Hello, Father. I've probably sinned. And probably need forgiveness. It's been from before birth since I did any kind of confession."

Before going to Haiti I listened to a CD on how to speak Haitian Creole and looked at the book that came with the tape, but I didn't learn very much. I'd had translators in Honduras. I've come to like having translators because there's a ritual and rhythm to it, and I get to watch mothers and children more closely while they're paying attention to the translator.

I saw a lot of deep, weeping chronic skin and scalp infections. I doubt that the ten days of antibiotics or antifungal medicine I was able to prescribe did much. We found out at the end of the trip that an as-yet-to-be-determined amount of the medications and other supplies we brought had been stolen. We also found out that our mildly depressed Haitian pharmacist was substituting medications she had for the ones she didn't. Thankfully, the clinic had full-time Haitian doctors, Haitian nurses, and Haitian community health workers to clean up after us. I'm resolved to go back and do a better job with lower cost and more sustainable answers to some of the problems we saw, especially the skin infections. Having an ongoing weekly wound-care clinic and teaching the community healthcare workers about bleach baths and gentian violet might be helpful.

I had no illusions that the thousand five-hundred-milligram amoxicillin capsules, ten cans of baby formula, and one case of Ensure that I stole from our office were going to do much, but it was better than nothing. Better than nothing is much appreciated in Haiti. When I go back, I'm bringing lots of cardboard books for the staff to give out to parents as part of well baby visits.

The Haitians were gracious and grateful for my efforts to speak Creole. I said "bon bagay" ("good thing") a lot, and "respire" ("take a breath"). I never thought my high school French would come in handy. I now harbor delusions that with practice I'll be able to speak Creole. The Haitians wanted us to do well and we did our best to live up to their expectations.

When I practiced pediatrics in Haiti and before in Honduras, I expected to see exotic and severe disease, but I was pleasantly surprised to learn that Haitian mothers, like mothers everywhere, worry about what their children eat and how they sleep. Haitians were willing to stand in line for hours to have the Yankee doctor tell them that vegetables don't matter much, some kids sleep a lot, others not so much, and that their child was beautiful and coming along well. Maybe I should have been saving life and limb, snatching children from the jaws of death, but there wasn't much life-and-limb work available.

The thing about having gone to medical school and completed a good residency was that I have an extra gear if I need it. At home and in Haiti, it's the extra gear that lets me enjoy doing my job. When I tell someone that their child doesn't have cancer or that they don't need an x-ray, they—not always but usually—take my word for it.

In the middle of a morning clinic, a couple from up the hill brought in a premature, delivered-at-home, barely breathing, less-than-six-months'-gestation, eyes-still-fused baby. I explained as best I could that the baby was much too early to live and got the priest.

The mother and father and some of the clinic staff couldn't stand the idea of not doing something and were gathering up what money they could to try to take the baby to a hospital. It cost about two hundred dollars cash up front to be admitted to the hospital; an unbelievably huge amount of money in Haiti. The baby died before reaching the hospital. I went up onto the roof deck and cried.

As in Honduras, the best thing about Haiti was being free of insurers rather than having to play the strange game of "Mother May I?" we've gotten used to playing back here at home.

At a medical clinic in Haiti or Boston Health Care for the Homeless or a free medical-care van, it becomes clear that we're all in this together: I want and need you to be immunized, get your diabetes and asthma well taken care of, get your drug habit under control, and wear a seatbelt.

There are plenty of people right here in the United States who are every bit as poor and lacking in access to care as the people of Haiti and Honduras. Giving away care is the ultimate way to improve access to care and to be in charge of what care is.

A well-trained doctor could set up a card table and a blood-pressure cuff in a church parking lot and do a lot of, or at least some, good. It would be a start. Better than nothing.

The Table Saw and the Thumb-- A Cautionary Tale

A year after going to Haiti, I cut off part of my thumb.

There's a very inexpensive notched plastic baby hockey-stick thingy called a push stick that's designed to keep thumbs and saw blades apart, and it usually works. I had actually bought one and was dutifully using it to saw a piece of walnut branch that fell in our backyard. Black walnut is beautiful and expensive wood. I wanted to see what the big deal was and if I could get anything useful from the fallen branch. I had about twenty minutes before I was supposed to be at work. Sometimes using things that are supposed to make life safer can make you overconfident.

The branch caught on something and stalled. My left thumb instinctively helped without consulting my brain, which was thinking about being at work in twenty minutes or so. The cut

187

through the walnut branch was finished straight and flush, along with a perfect forty-five-degree bisection of the terminal phalanx of my thumb. Table saws are so good at what they do that I noticed the blood before I realized where it all was coming from. Almost immediately I thought about how unnecessary the sawing of the walnut was (I could have just bought a block of goddamned walnut) and how many patients were going to have to be rescheduled. I didn't want patients to be rescheduled or ever know I'd cut off part of my thumb with a table saw.

It has been suggested that I'm accident prone. It has also been suggested that high utilizers of emergency rooms should pay higher co-payments, have higher deductibles, or both. This would be my fourth ER visit in ten years; not so bad.

Even with blood all over me and the presenting complaint of partial amputation of thumb, it took a while for me to be seen. My wife had gone back to the garage to look for the top of the severed thumb because the ER receptionist thought the surgeons might want it. She was unable to find it and was surprised to see my bloody-faced self still in the waiting area when she returned to the hospital. I had hoped that the blood, my being on the staff there, and my having taken care of their children might shorten the wait. Some of the staff know I live close by and called me once when a woman they were taking care of who was in a car crash went into labor. Babies, especially brand-new ones, make doctors who aren't used to them nervous.

My right hand was busy controlling the bleeding of my left hand so my wife did most of the paperwork. I had actually been able to get my wallet out of my shirt pocket, where she had put it. I retrieved my social-security Medicare card with my teeth.

"Oh, you've been here before," the front desk receptionist said.

X-rays and two Tylenol later, it came time to remove the gauze from my attenuated thumb. The pain was excruciating. Looking at the bill later, I saw that the Tylenol had cost Medicare nineteen dollars each. In our office we give Tylenol away for free. Thirty-eight dollars plus about 20 percent hospital and insurance administrative costs added about fifty dollars to the cost of everyone's medical care for something that cost less than ten dollars to make and that my wife could have brought with her on her way back from home if anyone had thought to ask her.

The Tylenol should have cost less, but with the hospital's sky-high overhead and tiny operating margins, they would have just had to find the thirty-eight dollars somewhere else. Shortly after my visit, the hospital was bought out by a healthcare conglomerate.

The medical-care and decision part of my ER visit took forty-seven seconds. "You're going to need a hand surgeon," said the ER guy, whose daughter I had taken care of. I had already guessed as much and could have saved time and money by going directly to the in-town hospital.

"Do you want to go by ambulance? Does anyone know where the other part of the thumb is? They might want to sew it back on."

My wife went back again to look, and my thirteen-year-old son again refused to help.

Hand surgery is a highly specialized field with five years of surgical residency training and then a fellowship. You have to really want to be a hand surgeon to become one. There are orthopedic hand-surgeon guys and plastic-surgery hand-surgeon guys. At MGH and most big ERs they take turns operating. My surgeon was one of the plastic-surgeon guys. They tend to be thinner and more thoughtful.

Had my surgeon decided that a skin graft, which would have made the hospital more money, was the way to go, that's what would have happened. Reattaching the severed part, if it had been found, would have coded even higher and made the hospital more money.

My surgeon was a happy man doing what he wanted to do. He chatted cheerfully about thumbs and fingers and table saws. It was a little deflating to learn how common my injury was. He talked some about different kinds of skin grafts, but in the end, he went with simple salt water, sterile gauze, frequent dressing changes, and narcotics.

"It's going to hurt," he said as he took off the gauze.

"Yikes," I said, but this time it hurt less than in the ER because he'd soaked my thumb in warm salt water first. What I got was standard Civil War treatment for partially amputated extremities, except that Civil War soldiers wouldn't have bothered seeking medical attention for such a minor injury.

"You'll able to do buttons again sooner if we don't do a skin graft."

My wife had to help dress me for a few months. I started wearing Western shirts with the shiny mother-of-pearl snaps.

For the wound checks, my surgeon would delicately unwrap the thumb as if he was dealing with nitroglycerin and admire how well it was coming along:

". . . you're granulating nicely. No signs of infection."

"Thanks."

There was virtually no pain with dressing changes after the first two weeks. The theatrically elaborate dressing and splint I wore to keep my thumb immobile made me look part mummy. It involved the whole hand and most of my forearm. I was on my way to see my hand surgeon for a wound check when a homeless guy I'd seen before on Blue Hill Avenue came up to my car window. I grabbed some quarters and was preparing to give them to him.

"What happened to your hand?"

"Table saw."

The homeless guy cringed as if he himself had just run his hand through a table saw. I gave him the quarters. For the next month or so, while my hand was wrapped in white cling-gauze wrap, almost everyone asked what had happened and then winced in empathetic pain when I said, "Table saw."

You can buy table saws with electronic sensors that can tell the difference between flesh and wood. When they detect flesh, they activate a braking mechanism that stops the whirring blade before it takes off body parts. There's an impressive demonstration of how it works on YouTube using a hot dog as a stand-in for your finger or thumb. The saw with the sensor costs extra. My wife and primary care doctor wonder why I haven't bought one and still have the same table saw that attacked my thumb.

"I've learned my lesson. It won't happen again," I promise.

Real carpenters show me their scars from encounters with saws, most of them more serious than mine.

"That's what we call a carpenter thumb, Doc. Ever shoot yourself with a nail gun?"

Marijuana is not your friend

> "Wow. Everything is so funny."
>
> ME, ca. 1968

The only thing dumber than making marijuana illegal is thinking it's harmless to children. There are people who can smoke a lot of pot without any ill effects. Your teenage years are not the best time to figure out whether you're one of them. Marijuana does different things to children than it does to adults. It also does very different things if you smoke it every day as opposed to once in a while. My highly prejudiced, unscientific point of view is that the fewer the once-in-a-whiles, the better.

Narcotics kill pain, physical and psychic. You and your brain can get some rest. Marijuana, on the other hand, kills the notion that there's anything that needs to be done.

Funny things happen when you're stoned. Sometimes everything is funny. The world and you slow down. Maybe you get arrested for driving too slow. You feel more a part of things as opposed to apart from things. Your friends are funny. The munchies are particularly funny.

Senses are heightened. Concerts and music are amazing. Everything is so amazing that you wish you could be stoned all the time. Ideas about what you should do tomorrow or after high school are laughably silly.

A few of my patients have medical marijuana cards. I doubt it's possible to see the marijuana doctor and not get a card. The marijuana doctor charges five hundred dollars for a five minute visit, doesn't use a stethoscope, and doesn't take insurance. I have one patient who stopped taking his bipolar meds because marijuana worked so much better. The results were not good. One day someone looked funny at his girlfriend. I don't know who actually started the fight, but my patient will be in prison for attempted murder for the foreseeable future. A large kitchen knife was involved. It's not marijuana's fault, but I don't have any patients for whom medical marijuana has worked out well.

"I'm really glad you got your card and are on medical marijuana" isn't something I've ever said or am likely to say. I haven't yet seen a case of anxiety, insomnia, or chronic pain that we don't have better treatments for.

I smoked pot as a teenager and in college. It's among many things I did as a teenager that I don't recommend. It was relatively weak, unavailable, and expensive. I wasn't a pothead and none of my friends were potheads. Stoners were rare.

I know of no other single drug, including alcohol and narcotics, that so thoroughly changes a kid's personality and ambitions. More than a few of my patients go from nonsmokers to daily smokers and it happens quickly, often over a few months. Among all the other funny things that happen, you can go to school stoned and nobody notices. Nobody cares. Except maybe your mother.

If you smoke every once in a while, your mother probably won't bring you to the pediatrician for a drug test. If you're a casual pot smoker, you won't talk about illegal search and seizure when your mother finds your not-very-well-hidden marijuana; you won't object strenuously to a drug test, saying it proves that your mother doesn't trust you. If you readily agree to the test, it might mean that you've come equipped with someone else's urine.

Sometimes I side with the patient.

"I agree with you that your mother should trust you. Your mother will trust you more if you agree to do a drug test in a month."

It's not a good sign if you can't clean up for a month to give clean urine. We also have a mouth swab test that they can't fake. Their faces fall when we tell them, "Great news, you don't have to pee in a cup. We're just going to swab your cheek."

If the cheek swab comes back positive, I say that it's probably a mistake. "Let's try again next month."

An ex-patient who's bringing her baby to us says, "Marijuana is legal and I have a medical card. Why is DSS [Department of Social Services] investigating me? Marijuana is legal. It's the grandmother who has it in for me. Marijuana is legal."

"Yeah. But if you can't give it a break for a little while I can see where DSS might be concerned."

I've known the grandmother for a long time. She comes to see me. She says she goes over to help out when she can, and tells me, "Kara doesn't even get up when Melanie cries. She feeds her but that's about it."

"But marijuana is legal."

The boy who could play anything

"Music is the only proof I need for the existence of God."

KURT VONNEGUT JR.

Aaron Gold was a saxophonist who took it upon himself to transcribe and play Coltrane and Thelonious Monk solos when he was seventeen. I admire Coltrane and Thelonious Monk and would play their music if I could. I've played rock-and-roll saxophone and tried to play jazz since I was eleven years old. At his annual physical I showed Aaron some pictures of me playing with an old rock band. He was more than a little depressed at the time and I suggested that maybe he would like being part of a band. Playing with a band feels fantastic—very different from and much better than playing along with CDs.

Septic Shock, "the world's best all-doctor rock band from MGH," which we started as interns, had small xeroxed posters in the halls advertising a pediatric-department party where we were playing. A senior cardiologist accosted me one day, saying, "There are patients in the hospital dying of septic shock. How do you think this makes their families feel?" I said to myself that they probably had other things on their mind. I shrugged pleasantly.

Most rock songs are simple enough that anyone who's ever played rock and roll can learn how to play them without much practice. I still play a little with one of the singer-guitarists from Septic Shock. I'm no Aaron Gold.

Aaron went to Berklee College of Music in Boston but wasn't very happy there. He switched to the New England Conservatory to study music theory and composition. He continued to come see me for medical care until he was twenty-three, when he moved to Chicago.

Several years earlier, when I was recovering from a psychotic break, I audited a music-theory course at Berklee and was lost in the dust after the first week. How could someone as talented as Aaron not succeed in the music world? I kept his immunizations up to date, treated his mild asthma, and continued encouraging him to start a band. He played some as a studio musician for a recording studio in Chicago.

One day his mother came to see me and told me that Aaron had jumped from the sixth floor of the building where he was living in Chicago. I felt a deep sense of loss for Aaron and the world. How could we not have taken better care of a kid so rare and so talented? There should be something like a monastery somewhere, where kids like Aaron can play music, have a small but regular allowance, and maybe have access to a cafeteria. Musicians like Aaron have already taken a vow of poverty and would be grateful for whatever help we can give them.

> *"Life is a fragile reed vibrating*
> *in the breath of God."*
>
> JOHN COLTRANE

Social media isn't social

"A dream you dream alone is only a dream. A dream you dream together is reality."
YOKO ONO

I've been talking to parents about a seriously sick child who happens to be theirs, when one of them stops me, "Excuse me," and reaches for the phone that just buzzed in their pocket. The "no cell phones in the exam rooms" signs we put up are constantly ignored. I've had one of my own doctors take a phone call in the middle of a physical exam.

When social media is an add-on to a busy life where you actually interact with other people in real time, there's nothing wrong with it, but if you go to sleep with your phone on the pillow and live for the phone to buzz, it's not good for you, especially if you're a teenage or preteen girl.

These days whenever there's a break at a medical conference or any other conference, 50 percent of the attendees whip out their phones. Some are just checking the news they've already checked three times that day and are trying to not look different or less important than everyone else. People used to talk to each other.

Calling is a step up from texting, because you hear someone's voice and inflections and how they respond to your voice, which transmits emotional information, but most young people text rather than call. If you want a call back, leave a voice message and you might get a text back. Young people are blindingly fast keyboarders even on the tiny screens on their phones.

Children notice whether their parents enjoy being parents and whether they themselves are important to their parents. It's hard for children to believe that they are important or that their parents are having a good time if they're compulsively checking their phones and responding to vibrations in their pockets.

Even if you have real and supportive relationships, the internet is a strange and potentially dangerous place where the lines between friend and predator are blurred. Teenagers really will destroy the GPS in their cell phones and get on a bus to meet up with a stranger they met on the internet, because it's a thing to do and they have no experience reading social cues.

"Friend" is not a verb. Virtual reality is not real. If you put the damn phone away, at least for meals, something good might happen. Tell your parents to do the same thing.

"Is it OK to break up by text?"

"No."

Psychiatrists by default

> "One is very crazy when one is in love."
> SIGMUND FREUD

Our patients with psychiatric problems used to be able to see psychiatrists. Now it's a six-month-plus wait, with formidable insurance hoops. So our seriously depressed, anxious, ADHD-afflicted, learning-disabled, self-harming, possibly psychotic, drug-addicted, alcoholic, and personality-disordered patients are stuck with us. Psychiatrists have been cheated out of their old job and forced to do three brief medication checks per hour now.

Primary care doctors do most of the diagnosing and treating of behavioral-health problems. We do a good job of it but it's not what we were trained to do or what we expected to be doing. Hiring social workers is the smartest thing I ever did. I recently hired a psychiatric medication nurse practitioner. These behavioral-health specialists help the rest of the practice function much more efficiently and happily. And when I have a patient who absolutely doesn't want to do therapy of any sort, I go get a therapist for them to talk to and explain why.

I expected and would have been perfectly happy mostly taking care of minor viral illnesses, doing my best to not miss curve balls, supporting parents, and helping them be the best parents they could be. I had to be honest and competent, but care is rarely about the disease or diseases we treat. Orthopedics isn't just about bones. Oncology isn't just about cancer. And pediatrics isn't just about "goo goo ga ga."

I have to be careful about the diagnosis I give, because what's in your medical record can be used against you. A record of ADHD, depression, anxiety, or asthma can make it complicated or impossible for a patient to become a cop or firefighter or soldier.

When possible, I use the "impulse control disorder" diagnosis. It's a real diagnosis with a real ICD 10 code.

Or "situational anxiety;" who doesn't have that?

Adjustment disorder?

Autism

> "What would happen if the autism gene was eliminated from the gene pool? You would have a bunch of people standing around in a cave, chatting and socializing and not getting anything done."
>
> TEMPLE GRANDIN, PH.D.

Danny was a fourteen-year-old autistic boy who had made remarkable progress, was making friends, and was doing well in school. When my youngest son, Oliver, was born, we put up notices in the office proclaiming the good news. Danny knew that I already had grown sons in their twenties. His father brought him in for an appointment and congratulated me on Oliver's birth.

"So what did you do with your first wife?" asked Danny. His father rolled his eyes.

The increase in the number of patients with autism is very real. It's not just being diagnosed more frequently, although that is going on too. When I started in practice, about one in a thousand children were autistic. We were maybe underdiagnosing autism, especially in high-functioning patients who had good receptive and expressive language skills. We were more likely to call them "atypical" children, or very shy or extremely introverted. We loved it when they did well, which they often did.

The root and tragedy of autism is how hard it is for autistic babies and kids to make connections with other people. It's especially hard and heartbreaking for their parents. It's about language, but it's more than that. Words without emotional content are better than no words, but the frustrations remain. There is no other therapy or therapeutic goal for autism beyond trying and trying and trying to make connection and make the child part of what we call "our world."

Babies come into this world looking for connection and milk. Shortly thereafter they start looking for identity and meaning, which are also about connection. They are free-floating probe vehicles looking for a way to hook up with something bigger than themselves. By four weeks, most babies are scanning for faces, and when they find one they smile and the face smiles back and they go berserk with joy. If you stick your tongue out, they can do that too. And they and you go to work reinforcing and tightening and locking their social-meaning probe to your social-meaning probe. And in a short period of time, you will do absolutely anything to protect and care for this baby and the baby fears nothing more than being separated from their people. And the mirroring goes on.

If I want a baby to like rather than fear me, which I do, all I have to do is notice arm or hand movements and imitate. The baby will be surprised at first but will eventually imitate my imitation. After a few rounds of "monkey see," we are usually friends. If I'm lucky I can perform an ear inspection without the baby's thrashing and screaming. Thrashing and screaming makes it hard for me to think straight. There are probably at least a dozen kinds of autism with a dozen or more causes, so now we call it autism spectrum disorder. I find lumping autistic patients together less helpful than separating them into categories and trying to figure out what works for which group. Lumping is lazy.

Babies like red, so I have a lot of red shirts. Who's programming who?

Danny had asked his question about my first wife as if he was a cop and I was a suspect. Maybe I had buried her in the backyard. He wanted to know.

"Good question, Danny. Sometimes things don't work out. You're good at math."

"I know."

Autistic boys greatly outnumber autistic girls. It's been suggested that autism is an extreme version of male social cluelessness. Girls learn to talk sooner and make friends earlier than boys and are better at both. These are also the two things autistic people have the most trouble with.

Quacks who claim to be able to treat autism and other poorly understood diseases—some of them made up—are now just as, if not more, prevalent than quacks of old. Quacks are often charismatic and always charming, as they champion their own "science" and lab tests and medications and procedures that "mainstream" medicine and science are trying to "suppress." When one of my families starts going down a quackish path, I tell them that to have an open mind is a good thing but to always keep their eyes open and one hand on their wallet. Keep an open mind but not so open that your brain falls out.

Most quacks are M.D.s. I'm unduly surprised by this and spend entirely too much time wondering if they believe their own claims. Why, after going through all the time and effort it takes to be a doctor, do they do exactly the opposite of what they were taught and trained to do?

What makes quackery increasingly attractive to patients and families is how pigheaded and inaccessible mainstream medical care has become. Quacks will at least talk to you, look at you when you talk, and return your phone calls.

If there's even a little connection, a little longing for meaning of any sort, it can be worked on. My favorite patients are autistic kids who have managed to make at least some connections. They are unique, invaluable people who continually amaze us. Honor-roll students and football-team captains are a dime a dozen.

How psychiatric medications and therapy work

"Is it peace or is it Prozac?"
CHERYL WHEELER

When people study ADHD, depression, anxiety, and other behavioral-health problems, what they usually find is that medication and therapy both work but that the best results come from using both together. We now have ADHD meds, antidepressants, anxiety medications, and other medications that work—not always, never perfectly, and not by themselves, but they work remarkably well compared to what we used to have.

All clinical encounters have common elements that are especially important when dealing with behavioral issues. Nearly all patients, whether depressed, anxious, or dealing with trauma, loss, divorce, ADHD, a mood disorder, or OCD, believe that they're unique, that there's nothing they or anyone else can do to help, that no one cares, and that their feelings and situation are permanent.

Merely coming to or being brought to a doctor for a behavioral problem means that someone cares—namely, the patient or the parent and, hopefully, the doctor. Clinical care, in and of itself, normalizes behavioral problems. And, maybe, the problem has a name, and other people have the same problem, and, unlikely but possible, the doctor's expertise might be useful and you might get better.

The important message at every step along the way is that someone cares and that others have had the same thing and recovered. Talk therapy and medication are more effective when used together. The positive effects of using both together are more than you would expect; it's more like multiplication than addition.

To some extent the same thing is true with so-called physical complaints. You might think that talking with someone wouldn't make antibiotics more effective or that a nice surgeon wouldn't have better results than a cold fish, but you would be wrong. When patients receive explanations from an empathetic, knowledgeable person, they are more likely to take medications and comply with other orders and suggestions. Both the physician's and the patient's positive expectations and mood, especially if the patient is discouraged or having difficulty paying attention, can be the difference between getting well and not getting well. The difference between infections and behavioral symptoms is that behavioral symptoms have a much longer, more complicated timeline: it's harder to tell when you're getting better.

The point of treating depression and anxiety is to make it possible for the patient to go out into the world and interact with other humans. To figure out how depressed patients are, ask them how their mood affects their life and what their friends think and how they're sleeping.

"Do you have friends? What do you guys do? How are you sleeping? What do you eat?"

The scariest thing for me as a doctor is the utterly flat,

unchanging affect of a patient who doesn't even smile at the possibility of getting a puppy.

It's important that there are things the patient can do to help the meds and therapy work better—walking two miles a day, eating well, decreasing social-media and screen time, taking care of a puppy, yoga, acupuncture, art, and music are all things that can help. Openness to trying potentially positive things, like openness to seeking help, is, in itself, empowering. The patient becomes sensitive to and aware of positive changes and those positive changes lead to more positive changes. What we hope to create is a positive spiral to counteract the negative spiral that's been pulling the patient down and into isolation.

Anyone who thinks that medication is the whole answer is their own kind of quack.

Everyone wants to sleep better, most people with behavioral issues don't sleep well. Even when you and a depressed or anxious patient can't agree on much else, you can agree that sleeping better would be a good thing.

"So let's work on that."

There is never nothing to do. Diet, exercise, writing down symptoms and what else was going on during any given day on a calendar, making yourself get up before eight a.m., taking a walk in the woods—these can all make a difference. You're not allowed to say they don't work unless you try them. If you're doing a bunch of things and feeling better, figuring out which are the key elements in the bunch and which aren't helping should be put off until later.

Increased serotonin is worthless if it doesn't translate into being able to talk to people and enjoy yourself, and do those other positive things like walking a few miles a day, eating better, avoiding social media, making some art, going out with real friends, doing yoga. Isolation is always the common denominator of any sickness. There's no healing without connection and if there's no caring, why bother?

> *"I did not know you could fracture the brain*
> *in your head and recover."*
>
> VINCENT VAN GOGH

✦   ✦   ✦

My own mental illness doubtless has a lot to do with why I've gravitated to behavioral-health issues and hired social workers. Having in-house social workers is relatively rare in primary care pediatric practices, but it makes the whole practice run more smoothly, even though it's only recently that we can bill for visits and that insurers will pay us for what our social workers do. In the beginning I could have cared less about how much money they brought in. I figured their presence and skill set would make the rest of the practice run more smoothly and I was right. Doctors make lousy social workers.

It's important that therapists and social workers have control over who they see and for how long. There are no productivity pressures for our therapists to bring in money. If their insurance doesn't pay, patients pay what they can on a sliding scale set by the therapist. I feel that my practice and I are getting away with something, to be able to do things this way. Our behavioral-health team lets our doctors do what they do best. We're able to do the right thing first and figure out how to pay for it second.

When I became acutely mentally ill and had to be hospitalized at the age of twenty-three, the doctors who took care of me believed in the

Medical Model. They taught me that there was no one to blame and nothing to be ashamed of. It was a biochemical screw-up; a disease like any other. Mental illness was no more creepy or mysterious than diabetes or asthma. It has never occurred to me to be embarrassed or ashamed about being mentally ill.

I've been worried about what others might think. I've been worried I might relapse or fail to recover. I've come very close to losing my profession. But I've never felt embarrassed.

"Stigma" is a dressed-up word for ignorance and prejudice. The stigma of mental illness makes it sound as if we're somehow marked and, further, that being marked limits our opportunities to get well and be part of society. In reality, there are no outward "marks." Most of us can and do clean up, dress up, and pass for normal.

My first hospitalization lasted about four months and cost about $12K. I was horrified that it was that high. The care was a long way from perfect, but the doctors and nurses took the time to talk to me, and not just once a day with a clipboard and a scribe. They helped me understand what the hell had happened to me, and that I could get better. Had I told them that I was going to write three books, go to medical school, and have three handsome sons, they would have upped my meds and taken away my day-room privileges.

The cost of not caring for the mentally ill dwarfs the cost of caring. The real pain and expense come from mental illness itself and what it does to families and patients.

There's no "mental" illness that doesn't include "physical" illness and vice versa. Even a simple ear infection can be the straw that breaks the camel's back.

The myth of mental wellness

> "Normal is just a setting on your dryer."
>
> PATSY CLAIRMONT

I occasionally give talks or write short articles for NAMI, the National Alliance on Mental Illness, a wonderful, chaotic grass-roots organization that helps patients and families find help and support.

It's crazy to expect people who haven't been mentally ill to act well. Expecting rational behavior, empathy, or helpfulness from others puts you in a dependent and usually uncomfortable position. Count on nothing but your own desire to be well. If you expect the worst, you may be pleasantly surprised. The bad behavior of others constitutes an "attractive nuisance" to someone recovering from mental illness. Your family might be suboptimal but so is everyone else's. Don't go swimming in that swimming pool; it's full of alligators. You need your energies, strength, and wits for things that matter.

A world without prejudice, stigma, or discrimination would

be a better world, but don't count on it or hold your breath. If recovery from mental illness depended on the goodness, mercy, and rational thoughts of others, then no one would get well. We're all cooked. Peace of mind, which we need more than anything else, is inversely proportional to our expectations.

Burnout

"When a veteran says he 'lost it,'
what did he lose?"
JONATHAN SHAY, author of *Achilles
in Vietnam*

Burnout is not just a matter of being overworked or being tired or not having enough time for hobbies and friends. Shorter work hours, long walks, and having a dog are good things, but doctors and nurses have been overworked and have been tired and have not had enough time for hobbies for generations. Burnout is treatable. Surviving combat fatigue and other forms of PTSD is a matter of feeling that you are not alone. You are not terminally unique. By talking and listening to each other's stories, burnt-out doctors and nurses become hopeful that their suffering can help others recover. The desire to be of service to others is both a reason and a way to get better.

Burnout is what happens to doctors and nurses who feel powerless and are unable to help patients. It's the feeling that one is a cog in a machine that doesn't care. Burnout makes people angry, depressed, and unable to do or enjoy doing the work of patient care. Burnout is loneliness, isolation, and an invitation to addiction, alcoholism, and other forms of self-harm. The biggest, most frequent and urgent question medical students ask when I give talks about mental health is "When do we get to help patients?"

A large part of how we came to be burnt out, and something generations of doctors and nurses who came before us rarely had to deal with, is the sense of betrayal and moral hazard. We're not exactly being ordered to napalm babies, but we are working harder and harder at jobs that seem less and less about helping people and more and more about making profits for CEOs who make $20 million to $50 million per year and for the insurance and the pharmaceutical industries. This isn't what we signed up for. Doctors are warriors who are waking up to find out that their leaders have betrayed them and given them unlawful orders and that there are a lot of dead civilians around.

There have always been depressed, anxious, alcoholic, drug-addicted, personality-disordered, obsessive-compulsive, neurotic, psychotic, suicidal, criminally insane, difficult-to-live-with, socially clueless doctors, but they were rarely burnt out.

Ninety-plus percent of what I used to do was clinical medicine; I diagnosed and treated disease. Now, half or more of what a hospital, a nurse, or a doctor does is redundant, worthless overhead that has nothing to do with taking care of patients. To the extent we can take good care of patients, we do so in spite of co-payments, quality improvement initiatives, and other unscientific, utterly ineffective, very expensive nonsense. When we do useful science, we do it in spite of blockbuster drugs and pharmaceutical share values and market caps. Not because of them.

Actually being in charge of care is an excellent and effective antidote to burnout. Turn the visit upside down by bringing the patient back to an exam room before collecting co-payments and verifying insurance. It's amazing what patients will tell you as you walk them down the hall. Do your own weights and vital signs.

Ask the patient what they're worried about and address their concerns. When you run out of things to talk about, the visit is over. Take them back up to the front desk, where they can do the insurance stuff.

If you're not attentive to patients and curious about their needs, you're not really caring for them and shouldn't bother being a doctor. Robots can do check lists and templates. Doctors and nurses shouldn't have to.

BURNOUT

Burn out is
being ordered to do worthless things or worse.
Having no choice or way out and being alone.
To have worked so hard for so long
to be a half million dollars in debt.
To be a replaceable
cog in a replaceable wheel,
doing mostly
data entry, click, click, clicking
into templated notes no one will ever read.
Is not what
I or anyone in their right mind would sign up for.
The medical endeavor has been stunned
into a breath-holding, glum quietness.
If you don't

like this job, you can be replaced, they say.

Where's my doctor?

say the patients.

I'll be with

you soon.

Has anyone verified

your insurance or reconciled your medication or

problem list?

I'm a zombie

and nobody cares.

It occurs to me:

maybe we are making our patients sick.

Maybe, like

washing our hands to prevent infections a hun-

dred-plus years ago,

we could figure out something to do about it.

Diabetics not

being able to afford insulin can't be right.

The real answer to the mystery of how Americans can spend so much on such bad medical care is that the amount of time and money being spent on patient care is far less than it used to be and less than it is in Europe and elsewhere.

Ulysses

> "There was never a genius without a touch of madness."
> ARISTOTLE

Ulysses was a god in my childhood. By the end of his life, he was just another guy in a nursing home dying of hepatitis C and liver failure; an addict who didn't do anything anymore except smoke weed and drink the occasional beer. He was never going to get the thousand-dollar pills or get onto a transplant list. He wouldn't have wanted all the fuss anyway.

Ulysses had been one of our town's two or three genuine juvenile delinquents. In the fifth grade, he knocked a teacher down the stairs when she tried to stop him from leaving in the middle of class. My response was that she shouldn't have gotten in the way. What good was going to come from getting in the way of a kid that fast and strong?

He was adopted. His parents had been told they couldn't have children. He and his adoptive father didn't get along even a little bit. His adoptive parents turned out to be able to have children after all and had two girls after they adopted Ulysses. It was said that, as a baby, Ulysses never cried or laughed and rarely smiled. When a baby never cries, it's not a good thing. It doesn't mean you're brave. It means that a baby has given up hope that there's any point in crying.

Ulysses was smarter, more athletic, and more talented than his father: much. When he was younger, it was mostly breaking windows and street lights. He had a very good arm and could hit windows from much further away than anyone else. I tried to break windows too but wasn't very good at it. But, once, on my first throw, I took out a street light.

Ulysses was olive skinned with black hair and eyebrows that met in the middle. He looked at least two years older than he was. It was generally conceded that Ulysses could beat up anyone his age and most, if not all, of the kids a grade or two above. He was exactly two years older than I was. We shared a birthday. He looked and probably was partly Greek, maybe a direct descendent of Plato or Hippocrates or Pythagoras.

When I was about ten, there was a birthday party that Ulysses wasn't invited to. Big mistake. Ulysses showed up anyway and beat us all up, but gently. It was more like a carnival ride than it was like a beating. Later, a Boy Scout troop started up and about a month into it we had an overnight camping trip on the tip of Sandy Neck, which was about two miles across the harbor. Ulysses was not part of the troop. Another mistake by the grown-ups involved. Ulysses took a skiff and rowed two miles across the harbor and then used that marvelous arm to lob beach rocks at our campsite. Two kids had to go to the emergency room to get stitched up, but no one was seriously hurt. Getting stitched up in a community hospital didn't cost much back then. Shortly after the camping trip the Boy Scout troop was dissolved. About all I remember learning in Boy Scouts was that paraffin-soaked cardboard was a good way to start a fire.

I wasn't used to being noticed or taken seriously much, but, for whatever reason, Ulysses started hanging out with me. He liked fishing, which was something I mostly did alone. He wanted to learn how to play chess, which I also knew how to do, though it wasn't exactly a popular pastime among my peers. I could still beat him but he learned lightning fast. Years later in high school when I was playing saxophone in a rock-and-roll band at the American Legion hall, Ulysses said he couldn't hear me and put the microphone directly into my saxophone so that you couldn't hear much else. "That's better," he said with a huge smile. Ulysses also played guitar better than anyone else around. He got us some jobs and was sort of our manager. Because he looked older than he was, he played with bands in twenty-one-and-older places and got to drink along with everyone else and pick up girls like everyone else and, eventually, do drugs like everyone else.

As a high school freshman, he tried out for football and became the starting quarterback, which thrilled his father. Ulysses and his father now had something to bond over, but it thrilled his father so much that Ulysses quit football and tried soccer, which his father did not care about. He was first-string all-state goalie that year. It goes on. Along with breaking the school record and winning the state track meet in javelin as a junior, he was playing semipro baseball when he was still in high school. The team lied about his age. He was right-handed with a perfect left-handed, Roger Maris-like swing.

He was a creature of habit and precision. When he pitched and I caught for him on a softball team, it was part of his rhythm and very important to him that I threw the ball back as close as possible to an exact spot a foot and a half to the left of his shoulder. Too low was the thing that threw him off the most. I did my best. When he was in his groove and on his game, he was virtually un-hittable. Once I threw out a guy at third and then got the game-winning hit the next inning. I had my moments.

I can't remember when exactly he taught himself how to play guitar. Maybe that was in high school too. He was playing and showing off within a year and I wondered if he had a brain as good as Mozart's. At dances at the American Legion hall and at local clubs, where he was too young to drink, he covered his left hand with a silk scarf so no one could steal his licks. He also did a thing where he fingered chords with his left hand while the drummer drummed on the steel strings.

When he was twenty, he was on a freighter with one of my cousin-brothers, on his way to Paris to try his luck as an expat musician, when his precious left hand got slammed in a door and was broken in several places. I think he would have made it in Paris, but who knows? He was good enough.

Adults, jealous of his looks and talent, seemed to think that his accident and failure to make it in Europe meant that reality was catching up with Ulysses; that he was an Icarus and had flown too close to the sun. Maybe he was. Maybe he was too talented to be allowed to succeed.

Just out of high school he'd been in a motor-scooter accident that broke his leg in two places, and he had to be operated on and hospitalized. Maybe he was given too much Demerol, but he didn't become an addict until years later. He fell off a ladder while working at The Cranberry Goose, an upscale touristy restaurant on 6A, and broke his leg again. He recovered and then fell again and broke the same leg, which had probably never quite healed.

Somewhere in there he became addicted to narcotics. He settled in on terpin hydrate, a cough medicine with codeine. It was plentiful, was barely addictive, and didn't set off alarm bells among pharmacists as he traveled up and down the Cape looking for the stuff. Like a lot of addicts, once he settled in to his addiction, he was a lot less trouble to the cops. He had traded in all his other problems and demons for the simple need to find narcotics.

Life got complicated and Ulysses fled to New Mexico where he worked at the Angel Fire ski area running the little-kid chairlift, making sure they got on OK and stopping the lift when they didn't. When he and I were both in our midforties, I took my two sons out to New Mexico for a February-break ski trip. It became important to me to track Ulysses down, even though the ski area where we were staying in Taos was at least an hour away from Angel Fire. He was amazed to see us, took us to the motel-like room where he lived, and kept saying how amazed he was that we had tracked him down. He asked whether we minded him smoking marijuana, which we didn't. He played his guitar and sang very spare Chuck Berry songs. No zillion notes and fancy chords as he used to play, no handkerchief on the left hand.

Two years after our visit, Ulysses came back to the Cape to help his son get sober. He never left the Cape and, to my knowledge, never crossed the bridge, which was true of many kids I knew growing up. There are Cape Codders who can achieve escape velocity and cross the bridge and those who can't.

As a child I was honored and, in a way, saved by Ulysses's friendship. It made me feel as if I was worth something, which is why I'm so pissed off that Ulysses was one of the many people who are allowed to sicken and die from hepatitis C without the benefit of those thousand-dollar pills that science meant to be for everyone.

If you're not going to treat Ulysses, who are you going to treat?

Erectile Dysfunction

Advertising is not the biggest part of what's gone wrong with medical care, but it's my favorite thing to hate and the clearest example of something that's good for profits and bad for patients and didn't used to be here and isn't found elsewhere in the world.

The pharmaceutical industry spent $6.5 billion on advertising last year, all of which was paid for by your insurance premiums, co-payments, and deductibles. Getting patients to ask for specific pills, buy specific insurance, or go to specific hospitals doesn't help anyone. If you're good, you don't have to trumpet it. If you're not good, trumpets, billboards, and marching bands won't help.

Science doesn't need promoting, but the medical journals where we learn about cutting-edge science are completely dependent on the twenty or more pages of shiny, full-color pharmaceutical ads they run in every copy. The cost of those ads is folded into the cost of unaffordable insulin and unaffordable everything else and co-payments.

I wish I could watch sports on TV without Viagra ads.

"Dad, what's erectile dysfunction?"

Along with pharmaceutical advertising, we have hospital and insurer advertising. "New and improved" used to be words we used to advertise soap.

"The World is Waiting"—

"Everyday Amazing"—

"Until Every Child is Well"—

"Innovative Models of Primary Care, Evidence-Based Translational Care, Quality-Improved, Data-Driven, High-Value, Provider-Incentivizing . . . transformative, value-based healthcare delivery."

Gag me.

Nowhere else in the world has the kind of ads that we do. Several billion dollars would be knocked off the cost of medical care if we went back to not allowing ads for prescription drugs on TV. We'd lose nothing and recoup $6.5 billion. Healthcare, which used to function more like the fire department, now looks like General Motors assembly lines, labor morale included. Ambulances used to be free.

It's not hard to connect the dots. Medical journals, even the honest ones, are utterly dependent on pharmaceutical advertisements. The science in these ads is only slightly more credible than that of the erectile-dysfunction ads on TV. Even if the pharmaceutical industry rarely, if ever, attempts to influence journal content, articles critical of the industry are few and far between. Articles that directly or indirectly blame patients, doctors, and nurses for the high cost of care are much more common.

Much of the vaccine refusal I deal with every day comes from how much of medical care has become unseemly, unscientific, disingenuous, money-driven bullshit. It would help if doctors and nurses publicly took a stand against drug-company ads and quackery as we did a hundred years ago. Part of our job as doctors should be to protect our patients from profiteers just as we protect them from infections.

Our profession and the general public are numb. My teachers are rolling over in their graves. We are using the same methods and often exactly the same words that quacks and charlatans used to sell sugar pills, revitalizing tonics, and goat testicles. We should truly be ashamed and not so puzzled about why the public doesn't respect and trust us the way they used to.

The Zombie Apocalypse

Staffing levels and support services used to be determined by nurses and doctors, who said what they needed. Administrators made sure they got it, and insurers, with a minimum of administrative overhead, paid for it. Care was more efficient, doctors and nurses and patients were happier, and healthcare cost a fraction of what it does today.

"The doctor won't see you now" and "Your nurse is busy" are not what patients who need care should be hearing. Long waits make people pissed off and harder to diagnose. Patients are more and more convinced that they don't matter to doctors.

A burnt-out doctor or nurse, like someone with 104-degree fever and the flu, should probably not be working with patients, but they usually can't afford to stay home.

Welcome to Zombie Healthcare.

Single-payer healthcare would make paying for our care much

less complicated. There is more support for single-payer health-care than ever before, but it's still a politically fraught question that the insurance industry—with their vast financial resources, lobbyists, and members of Congress—has successfully resisted for decades and might well be able to resist for years to come.

Unfortunately, it would be possible to end up with a single payer paying for underfunded, lousy zombie healthcare. If insurers successfully insist on having their interests protected and drug companies do the same there won't be much money left over for patients, nurses, and doctors.

The key to affordable quality healthcare is putting doctors and nurses back in charge. Duh.

COVID-19

Medical science is complicated. The mission is not. During COVID-19 we've had to function like battlefield medics, taking care of casualties without regard to rank or insurance status. Co-payments, prior authorizations, and deductibles have been suspended. Hospitals are sharing resources and information. Researchers are sharing research. Be it a bomb, a fire, or a pandemic, responding to emergencies is a critical part of what healthcare workers do. We improvise and expand access to care to see whoever needs to be seen. We don't go home at five.

COVID-19 presents us with a chance to change healthcare from the money-driven enterprise it's become back to something we can all be proud of and that serves the needs of everyone. The details of how patients are treated should be determined by doctors and nurses in accord with science. It's not complicated.

Healthcare workers should not let themselves be dragged back into a world where treatments, vaccines, and phone calls will be available to some people but not others.

Job one is to always take the best care we can of individual patients, which in turn is the best way to care for public morale and health. Figuring out how to pay for the care involved doesn't matter much in an emergency. Caring for patients with COVID-19 has been expensive, but not caring would be even more expensive. Taking care of patients is what we went to school for. Unfortunately, COVID-19 survivors and their families are already getting outrageous bills they can't possibly pay.

We are all in this together as surely as if the planet were being invaded by aliens. We should fight like banshees to hold on to rediscovered common values and common interests. If we can do that, we will return to our roots and much of our current discontent with medical care could go away.

Hospitals that a couple of months earlier were beating each other's brains out maneuvering for market share and enhanced reimbursement are now cooperating. Doctors and nurses were called out of retirement. We would have done better if so many hospitals hadn't gone out of business or if there weren't so many and such severe economic and healthcare disparities. Masks and PPE would have helped. Better housing, education, healthcare, and economic opportunities would have helped more. Healthcare disparities are at the root of why we did so much worse with COVID-19 than anyone else did.

Healthcare is not a finite exhaustible resource. It can expand to meet the challenges. Over the past forty years we've made healthcare an artificially expensive, scarce resource. We now have case managers, utilization reviewers, and other gatekeepers to keep out the riffraff. We have to remember that ultimately patients pay for everything and should have a say in how health-care gets paid for.

Along with setting up tents, military-hospital ships, and other temporary facilities and bringing medical residents in training on board, we increased access to care by dropping some of the usual gatekeeping. While coinsurance for COVID-19 might seem a minor detail, it has actually saved patients and their families hundreds of millions of dollars. Delivering healthcare for less money is a big part of what patients want and is something we can do and should be doing.

There was a time when all you needed to get insulin was to have diabetes; we wiped out polio for nickels and dimes (literally) and figured out how to cure leukemia for not much more. Science and medical care are living things that have to be used to stay alive. Either we practice medical care or we lose it.

Once upon a time, the patient was king. Doctors believed in science. They used science to discover what was true and what was not, in the service of making the king's life better. Doctors who did a lousy job were fired by the king.

As it did in the beginning, science will do its best to tell us what's true and what's not. Caring about and for patients has never been easy, but it's truly all there is.

OPTIMISM

I said in the beginning that I was an optimist. I believe we can and will get to a place where we take better care of patients. I believe that how we get there is relatively simple: procedures and practices that hurt patients should not be part of medical practice.

We now have plenty of evidence that co-payments and deductibles cause significant harm. In one study there was a 34-percent increase in mortality attributable to co-payments for prescription medications. It's not surprising that not being able to afford prescribed medications is bad for you. Most doctors and most patients most of the time know what they are doing and it is unlikely that making care more expensive would improve the quality of care.

Co-payments and most other innovations in healthcare delivery are intended to eliminate unnecessary care by incentivizing patients to be more careful consumers and incentivizing doctors to be more careful providers. There actually are ways to eliminate unnecessary care, improve the value and quality of medical care, and control costs that work. Patients and doctors are already highly incentivized to avoid unnecessary care. Not surprisingly, putting patients, nurses, and doctors back in charge of patient care, along with increasing the resources devoted to clinical care, increases the value and quality of care. This is not new. It's how things used to be done, but the problem is that many of the expensive, unnecessary, harmful practices we need to deal with are profitable for insurers.

The same hepatitis A, B, and C, HIV, TB, mental illness, and addiction currently living under bridges in the homeless population will eventually find their way into gated communities. We are all in this together. We all benefit when patients get prompt high-quality care for COVID-19 and whatever else comes our way.

Gatekeeping has never worked even a little bit and has nearly always made high- and low-value care more expensive. Gatekeeping has dramatically increased hospital- and office-practice overhead and has never decreased unnecessary care or lowered costs.

Do no harm. We don't approve new medications or medical devices without knowing, for sure, that they help patients more than they hurt them. Insurers and innovations in healthcare delivery should be held to the same standards. There's no question that patients trust us less than they used to. Being trusted and being trustworthy are absolutely essential to the practice of medicine. Without trust, it's next to impossible to practice good medicine and absolutely impossible to enjoy it. To the extent that what we do is dominated by direct and indirect pressure to meet metrics and other nonsense, why should patients trust us? Why should they take us seriously? Why wouldn't we get depressed?

The "we can do more with less" enthusiasts ignore the inherent and unavoidable conflict of interest between patients and insurers. Co-payments and denials of coverage work well for payers but badly for patients, always. Lowering co-payments, deductibles, and the cost of health insurance increases the quality and value of healthcare, always. It's like finding gold at the end of the rainbow.

Most people believe that having patients pay for more of their own care and having insurers deny care is bad for the individuals involved, but it keeps costs down for the rest of us: this is 100 percent wrong. Insurers are in the business of making money, which isn't evil but works out particularly badly in healthcare. The money insurers make from co-payments or not paying claims is legally theirs. They are under no obligation to share these proceeds with patients, doctors, or hospitals. Another issue is that not paying for or providing healthcare makes sick people sicker, which has significant adverse individual- and public-health consequences. When we don't pay for necessary care we are re-creating the diseases we've spent the last two hundred years learning how to treat effectively. Last but not least, 90-plus percent of us will need healthcare at some point. It would be nice to have the care you need be accessible and affordable when that day comes. Two-thousand-dollar ambulance rides, ten-thousand-dollar ER visits, and hundred-thousand-dollar operations are not good for you or anyone else.

We don't need new metrics, balancing acts, leaps of faith, or models of healthcare delivery. Roughly half of what we spend in the name of medical care is unnecessary and could be done away with. Wrangling about money has nothing to do with taking care of patients.

Another way to look at our cost and quality problems is one of lost patient autonomy and power. Doctors and nurses are trained, highly motivated patient advocates. There are virtually zero instances where having insurers tell patients, doctors, and nurses what to do results in better or less expensive healthcare. There are patients and providers who are hell-bent on greed, quackery, or just plain useless care. Unfortunately, co-payments, QI, and performance metrics don't slow them down or dissuade such patients and doctors even a little. Sometimes an empathetic nurse or doctor can talk sense into them. We could have and should have guessed that having insurers, rather than patients, nurses and doctors, in charge wouldn't end well. We don't do the job perfectly, but we do it well enough that insurers don't help us do it better.

We've spent thousands of years learning how to practice medicine. Not caring for ourselves or others is not, never has been, and never will be the smart way to go. It's not left, right, or center; it's math.

The needs and interests of patients have to come first. Always.

The End

ACKNOWLEDGMENTS

My wife is the most wonderful editor ever.

ABOUT THE AUTHOR

After writing *The Eden Express*, a memoir detailing his struggle with mental illness, Mark Vonnegut went to Harvard Medical School. He lives with his wife and son in Milton, Massachusetts, where he continues to practice primary care pediatrics. His most recent book is *Just Like Someone without Mental Illness Only More So* (Delacorte Press 2010).